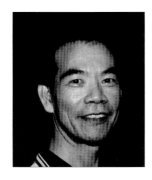

Dr Paul Lam, MBBS, FAMAC, a family physician and tai chi master in Sydney, Australia, for thirty-two years, is a world leader in the field of tai chi for health improvement. He has published widely in medical journals and magazines and is author of *Overcoming Arthritis*, *Tai Chi for Beginners and the 24 Forms* and *Teaching Tai Chi Effectively*.

Dr Lam has worked with tai chi and medical specialists to create several tai chi for health programs — including Tai Chi for Diabetes — that are safe and easy to learn. Dr Lam has travelled around the world training thousands of Tai Chi for health instructors.

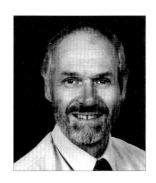

Dr Pat Phillips, MBBS, MA(Oxon), FRACP, MRACMA,GRADDIP HLTH ECON (UNE), is the Senior Director of Endocrinology at the Central Northern Adelaide Health Service. He has been actively involved in Diabetes Australia, the Australian Diabetes Society and the Australian Diabetes Educators' Association since the 1980s. He is an editor of the *Australian Guidelines for the Management of Diabetes in General Practice* and of Diabetes Australia's national diabetes magazine *Conquest*. He oversees the Diabetes Centre at The Queen Elizabeth Hospital and the State Diabetes Outreach Program.

TAI CHI FOR DIABETES

LIVING WELL WITH DIABETES

DR PAUL LAM & DR PAT PHILLIPS

ROCKPOOL
PUBLISHING

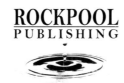

A Rockpool book
Published by Rockpool Publishing
1/2 Cooper Street, Double Bay, NSW 2028, Australia
www.rockpoolpublishing.com.au

First published in 2008

National Library of Australia
Cataloguing-in-Publication Entry

Lam, Paul.

> Tai chi for diabetes / authors, Paul Lam ; Pat Phillips.
> Sydney : Rockpool Publishing, 2008.
> ISBN: 9781921295140 (pbk.)

> Tai chi. Diabetes--Exercise therapy. Diabetes--Alternative treatment.
> Self-care, Health.

> Phillips, Pat.
> 613.7148

Cover and internal design by Seymour Designs
Typeset by Anthony Bushelle Graphics
Printed and bound by Everbest Printing Co
10 9 8 7 6 5 4 3 2 1

Contents

Foreword

The health benefits of tai chi are widely recognised. With more people living with diabetes who would benefit from all types of exercise, we encourage people with diabetes to participate in this low-impact sport.

Diabetes Australia supports physical activity as an integral part of managing diabetes. It can be challenging for people with diabetes to find a suitable activity and participate in exercise regularly. Turning diabetes around can start with incorporating physical activity into your lifestyle every day. Tai chi may provide that opportunity for you.

Dr Paul Lam is a practicing physician and well-recognised tai chi expert. Dr Pat Phillips is the Senior Director of Endocrinology at the Central Northern Adelaide Health Service. He has been caring for people with diabetes since 1987, through his work as a dedicated endocrinologist and as editor-in-chief of *Conquest*, Diabetes Australia's official magazine.

In this book, Dr Lam and Dr Phillips have combined their expertise to bring the reader both an easy-to-learn tai chi program and comprehensive information on diabetes.

Over the years, the Tai Chi for Diabetes program has helped many people with diabetes. I hope you will try it, with some wonderful results.

— Dr Gary Deed
President, Diabetes Australia

Prologue

In 2000 one in four adult Australians had abnormal glucose metabolism, the equivalent of the adult population of Melbourne. About 200,000 New Zealanders, nearly 18 million Americans, 2 million Canadians have diabetes. And worldwide, diabetes is a more serious health problem than HIV/AIDS. Recent WHO calculations indicate that almost 3 million deaths per year are attributable to diabetes.

Why is this epidemic happening? What can we do to stop it?

The three major risk factors for diabetes are: increasing age (over forty), diabetes in the family (family history) and overweight (fatness) — what we call 'the three Fs'. Changes in two of these risk factors are responsible for the epidemic: in Western countries around the world there is an increase in the number of people over forty and a lot more of us are overweight and inactive.

This book is about how you can reduce your diabetes risk if you don't have diabetes — and, if you do have it, how you might overcome diabetes. Several studies have shown that if you change the way you live, your body will work better, you will feel better and you'll enjoy life more.

Tai chi, the ancient Chinese exercise/art, can help to prevent and improve the control of diabetes. This book features step-by-step instructions, illustrated with photos, of each movement of the specially designed Tai Chi for Diabetes program.

Although Tai Chi for Diabetes is designed for people with diabetes, you don't have to have diabetes to use the tai chi program. It's excellent exercise for relaxing, improving your health and for a better quality of life. And studies have shown that gentle exercise and a healthy diet can actually *prevent* people from developing type 2 diabetes.

If you are a health professional, you can recommend the tai chi program as an exercise for patients. In addition, you'll find the information and resources provided helpful in your care of people with diabetes.

How to use this book

The book is in three sections. Part I provides information about diabetes and how to manage the condition so that you can enjoy a better quality of life. Part II consists of the Tai Chi for Diabetes program — if you lean more towards 'doing', you can simply read the introductions to each section and then start straight into the program. Later on, you can go back to more in-depth reading about the background of tai chi. Part III is a list of useful resources to help you live well with your condition.

As a tai chi beginner, you can use this book by itself or in conjunction with classes and/or the instructional *Tai Chi for Diabetes* DVD. Be sure to consult your health professional about the program and how to make adjustments, according to your own ability and requirements. If you don't have an instructor, please follow the instructions and progress steadily. Learning a lot of tai chi movements quickly doesn't necessarily give you greater benefit or more satisfaction. Steady and careful progression does. You must read chapter 4, Getting Ready, before starting so that you understand how to do the program safely and effectively.

Tai chi is a different type of exercise from most Western sports. The emphasis is on slowness and being mindful, and its movements follow a circular path instead of a straight line. Most people need time to get used to these concepts. Be patient with yourself and give yourself time to learn each segment well before moving on to the next one. You will enjoy the program more and gain much more benefit doing it naturally and steadily — the tai chi way.

A note for tai chi teachers

The book is useful as a reference for you to understand the condition of diabetes and how to teach the program safely and effectively. We suggest you read all chapters in the sequence presented to gain a good understanding of the condition and the Tai Chi for Diabetes program. If you have not already done so, we strongly recommend you attend the instructors' training workshop with Dr Lam or his authorised master trainers so that you learn the most effective way to teach the program safely.

PART I

CHAPTER 1

DIABETES EXPLAINED

What is diabetes?

Diabetes occurs when there is insufficient insulin to enable the body to use glucose normally.

There are three main types of diabetes:

- type 1, when the body does not produce insulin
- type 2, when the body makes insufficient insulin or does not use the insulin it does produce efficiently
- gestational, which occurs during pregnancy when the amount of insulin required increases and the body can't supply enough.

Type 1 diabetes may be associated with other immune conditions affecting the thyroid, the lining of the intestine (coeliac disease) and the stomach (gastritis, pernicious anaemia).

Type 2 diabetes may be associated with high blood pressure, high blood fats and a tendency to clot. In women, polycystic ovary syndrome (irregular periods, lowered fertility) may precede diabetes.

Diabetes: what goes wrong?

Diabetes was known in ancient times. The disease's full name, *Diabetes mellitus*, comes from the Greek. *Diabetes* — *dia* meaning 'through' and *betes* 'a passing' — refers to the passing through the body of large volumes of fluid. *Mellitus* means 'honey'. The name captures the basic problem in diabetes: the sweetness of the urine and other body fluids caused by too much sugar.

Your body needs a special sugar, which is called *glucose*. The body makes glucose from starchy foods — carbohydrates such as bread and potatoes — and from other sugars — for example, from sucrose (table sugar) or fructose (the sugar contained in fruit). The glucose is carried around the body in the blood: the level of glucose in the blood is called *glycaemia*.

A question of balance

Blood glucose can be controlled by balancing the things that increase glucose levels (food, stress) with those that decrease blood glucose (activity, medication).

Your glucose level must be neither too high nor too low … but just right.

A high level, called *hyperglycaemia*, affects the body's machinery. Things don't work as well:

- You feel tired and sleepy.
- The body fluids are out of balance because of the high levels of glucose.
- The lens in your eye changes shape and you get blurry vision.
- The kidneys filtering the blood collect more glucose than usual. Because this glucose must be carried out of the body, you pass a lot of urine (polyuria); therefore, you need more water, get thirsty and drink a lot (polydipsia).
- Your body loses glucose from food products. Consequently, you lose weight, feel hungry and eat more (polyphagia).

A low glucose level, known as *hypoglycaemia*, also affects the body, especially the brain which relies on glucose. Your brain doesn't like being starved of glucose. It sends urgent signals to the body:

- You feel hungry.
- You don't think straight.
- You get trembly.

WHAT'S IN A NAME?

Many of the names we use for parts of the body, diseases and conditions were given by Greek physicians over two millennia ago:

Diabetes mellitus: *dia* = through, *betes* = a passing, *mellitus* = honey

Glycaemia: *glyc* = glucose, *aemia* = in the blood

Hyperglycaemia: *hyper* = high, *glyc* = glucose, *aemia* = in the blood

Hypoglycaemia: *hypo* = low, *glyc* = glucose, *aemia* = in the blood

Polyuria: *poly* = lots, *uria* = urine

Polydipsia: *poly* = lots, *dipsia* = drink

Polyphagia: *poly* = lots, *phagia* = to eat

Where does glucose come from?

The meals you eat include: *protein* — for body growth and repair; *fat* — which has lots of concentrated calories, and *carbohydrates* — in starchy foods and sugars. Each is made up of simple units.

Starch, which has hundreds of smaller units joined together, is a *complex carbohydrate*. The small units in starch are sugars, such as glucose and fructose; they are *simple carbohydrates*.

Food is broken down by digestive juices. Starch is digested into sugars, which the liver makes into glucose. Your body can't change straw into gold (remember the fairytale of Rumpelstiltskin) — but it can change bread into glucose.

Insulin enters the story

The starch has been turned into glucose, which is racing around in the blood stream. But the glucose has to get out of the blood and into the body tissues. This work is done by the cells in the body tissues: brain cells — so you can think; heart cells — so your blood can pump; muscle cells — so you can walk.

But these cells require a trigger. Insulin opens the doors — the glucose channels — that let glucose go from the blood to the body cells.

Insulin comes from the pancreas, a gland sitting just below the stomach, halfway between your belly button and the imaginary line joining your nipples. Most of the cells of the pancreas make digestive juices, but some cells (the beta cells) make insulin, which travels in the blood and tells the food products where to go.

Maintaining the balance

Your body is very clever. A high blood-glucose level makes the pancreas produce more insulin. Insulin opens the glucose channels and glucose flows from the blood into the cells. The blood glucose falls and the body gets back into balance.

At rest, the cells don't need much glucose. The glucose channels are difficult to open as there is not much insulin present.

After a meal containing starch, blood glucose increases: the pancreas releases insulin, which opens the glucose channels and the cells use the glucose.

When exercising, the muscle cells need glucose. There is not much insulin, but the demand for glucose by the cells stimulates and opens up the glucose channels and allows glucose through.

In diabetes, insulin levels are decreased or the insulin produced does not work properly. Glucose channels are shut. This means that glucose builds up in the blood and causes problems.

The balancing act

The aim of diabetes treatment is to keep the blood glucose balanced in the normal range — because this is no longer being done automatically by the body. People with diabetes must organise and juggle food and stress, insulin and/or tablets, and exercise. What have to be balanced are:

- the things that raise blood glucose — food and stress
- the things that lower blood glucose — exercise and insulin/tablets.

If this balancing act is successful, blood glucose doesn't get too high (hyperglycaemia), or too low (hypoglycaemia), but stays in the healthy range.

Highs and lows

Glucose levels go up and down throughout the day.

High blood glucose occurs about two hours after meals and when you are under stress.

Low blood glucose occurs before meals, after exercise, sometimes in the middle of the night and other times when there is a long gap between meals.

What are you aiming for?

The basic problem with diabetes is that the blood-glucose level rises. This abnormal chemistry can damage the body. Therefore, it is important to control blood glucose to avoid problems.

Everyone is different. You and your healthcare team will work out your own personal goals. In a perfect world, we would aim at the levels that occur in people without diabetes because we believe that this minimises long-term problems. Often though, it is impossible to get this ideal control, and trying too hard can cause blood glucose to swing from high to low. It is a question of finding the balance that suits you best.

The types of diabetes

The basic cause of diabetes is the same: not enough insulin action to control metabolism. However, there are three main forms of diabetes.

CHARACTERISTICS OF TYPE 1 DIABETES

Previously known as insulin dependent diabetes. It usually develops in young people.

Who is affected? Usually children and people under thirty. Often there is no family history of diabetes.

What goes wrong? No insulin is produced by the pancreas.

Onset Symptoms occur suddenly and severely (days to weeks). People often present with excessive thirst, passing urine frequently, loss of weight and tiredness. Sometimes they lose consciousness.

Treatment Insulin injections as well as healthy nutrition, exercise and a healthy lifestyle.

Type 1

In type 1 diabetes the body's immune system doesn't recognise the cells that make insulin (beta cells) in the pancreas. Instead, it treats them as though they are foreign and destroys them.

The immune system may also not recognise other parts of the body and destroy these as well. This is more common in people with type 1 diabetes and it particularly affects the thyroid gland (causing over- or under-activity) and the lining of the gut (causing poor food absorption, coeliac disease, inflammation, poor absorption of vitamin B12 and pernicious anaemia).

If other family members have type 1 diabetes and/or have had problems with their thyroid, coeliac disease or pernicious anaemia, you may wish to check your risk. Your doctor can arrange a blood test that looks for markers of immune destruction (antibodies), which can indicate that you may develop one or more of these problems.

Type 1 diabetes usually develops suddenly without any obvious warning. Those affected are often young people, have an excessive thirst and need to urinate frequently.

Type 1 diabetes must be treated with the utmost seriousness. At present, insulin injections are the only known treatment. However, with proper treatment and care, many people with type 1 diabetes lead normal and productive lives. Good management — insulin combined with exercise and a healthy diet — is based on maintaining the blood glucose in the normal range.

New developments are on the horizon. One example is a small apparatus that works almost like an artificial pancreas and can be implanted under the skin. Insulin can also be delivered by nasal spray instead of by injection.

The Tai Chi for Diabetes program is suitable for those with type 1 diabetes. Before beginning the program, you should discuss it with your health professionals.

CHARACTERISTICS OF TYPE 2 DIABETES

Usually develops in older people and is also known as non-insulin dependent diabetes.

Who is affected? Usually affects those over fifty years of age and who are overweight. A family history of diabetes is common.

What goes wrong? Some insulin is produced but is not effective or only partially effective.

Onset Symptoms occur more gradually (weeks to months, even years). Sometimes there are no symptoms. Half the people with type 2 diabetes are undiagnosed.

Treatment Often controlled by healthy nutrition, exercise and a healthy lifestyle. May need tablets or insulin in some cases.

Type 2

In type 2 diabetes the body is resistant to insulin and the pancreas can't make enough to overcome this resistance.

Type 2 diabetes is often associated with excess weight around and in the abdomen. This sort of fat distribution may be associated with other problems, particularly high blood pressure, high blood fats and a tendency for the blood to clot. Some women who have had irregular periods or problems conceiving children may also have cysts on their ovaries (polycystic ovary syndrome) and later develop type 2 diabetes.

If you have type 2 diabetes, you are more likely to have clotting of your blood vessels: your blood pressure and blood fats will need to be checked regularly and your doctor will advise on appropriate treatment to reduce any tendency of the blood to clot. If you have had polycystic ovary syndrome, you are more likely to develop diabetes, so please ask your doctor to check your blood glucose every year or so.

Type 2 is by far the most common diabetes. About 90 per cent of people with diabetes have this type. Usually slow in onset, type 2 used to be called 'maturity onset diabetes', because it mainly affects people over fifty.

In this type of diabetes, either the body is not producing enough insulin or the insulin produced is not as effective as it should be. It is caused by an unhealthy lifestyle — lack of physical activity and an unhealthy diet — and genetic predisposition. Unfortunately, in recent years more young people are being affected by this condition, and this can be attributed to an unhealthy lifestyle. The disease is largely preventable with a good diet and gentle exercise.

Many people with type 2 diabetes often don't know that they have it because there are no symptoms until the disease has reached the advanced stages. Early detection and treatment is essential to prevent significant and irreversible damage to the body, so have regular medical check-ups.

Exercise and diet are the cornerstones of treatment. Approximately 50 per cent of people with type 2 diabetes are initially treated successfully with better diet and regular exercise and do not require medication. Other treatments include oral medication and insulin injection.

The Tai Chi for Diabetes program is suitable for people with type 2 diabetes, but check with your doctor first.

Gestational

Gestational diabetes is a type of diabetes that develops during pregnancy. It usually occurs around the middle of the pregnancy and affects about 3 per cent of pregnant women.

During pregnancy the body produces many different kinds of hormones. These hormones can block the action of insulin in the body, causing 'insulin resistance'. In gestational diabetes there are high levels of glucose in the bloodstream.

It has been found that the likelihood of developing gestational diabetes is increased for those who:

- have had gestational diabetes previously
- have a family history of diabetes
- are over thirty years of age
- are overweight
- have had 'large' babies (over 4 kg)
- have had unexplained stillbirths or miscarriages.

Gestational diabetes usually goes away after the birth. However, it is very important to continue to be tested for diabetes every year after the delivery, and before stopping contraception and trying to become pregnant again. This is because women who have developed gestational diabetes have a high risk of developing type 2 diabetes.

Other related conditions

Pre-diabetes

Also known as impaired glucose tolerance and impaired fasting glucose. In this condition, people have abnormally high blood sugar, but it is not high enough to be classified as diabetes.

People with pre-diabetes are likely to develop type 2 diabetes in five to ten years time unless preventive measures are taken. Gentle exercise and a healthy diet can prevent diabetes from occurring in about 60 per cent of those diagnosed with pre-diabetes.

Estimates show that between 1988 and 1994, 40.1 per cent of the American population aged between forty and seventy-four had pre-diabetes. Around two million Australians had pre-diabetes in 2004.

Why do we get diabetes?

It is not known exactly how people get type 1 diabetes. It is not clear why the body's immune system doesn't recognise the beta cells that make insulin in the pancreas, treats them as if they are foreign and destroys them. Type 2 diabetes is mainly caused by an unhealthy lifestyle.

Can you prevent diabetes?

We know that people who are less active are more likely to develop diabetes. Many scientific studies have shown that diet and exercise can prevent diabetes. In overweight people, the loss of 5 to 10 kilograms of weight in a year, together with regular gentle exercise, has been shown to reduce the risk of developing type 2 diabetes by about 60 per cent.

Tai chi is a gentle exercise with a strong emphasis on mental relaxation. It can also help prevent diabetes. One of the problems with exercise is that most people don't stick to it regularly. The Tai Chi for Diabetes program is designed to be enjoyable and has a higher rate of adherence — many people continue to practice it for years.

If we don't like doing something or if we don't do it well, we tend not to do it at all. That's often true of exercise. People who are not well coordinated tend to perform badly in sport, and therefore they are less likely to enjoy it. Imagine a man who's poorly coordinated and walks with a little clumsiness. Perhaps from childhood, people have made fun of the way he walks. It is quite likely he would unconsciously minimise walking to avoid being laughed at. Likewise with other activities and sports.

In our experience, many people with diabetes are less interested in and less likely to adhere to an exercise regime. Tai Chi for Diabetes is designed to improve coordination and can be learned relatively quickly. By exercising regularly, there will be significantly less chance of developing diabetes. See chapter 4, Getting Ready, which provides guides on how to start and how to keep going.

Health challenges for diabetics

Potential long-term problems of diabetes

The major goal of diabetes treatment is to delay or prevent problems and complications that can result from high or low blood-glucose levels. Some problems can occur suddenly, such as hyperglycaemia or hypoglycaemia (see pages 3–4).

Frequent high blood-glucose levels damage the body. The areas most affected are the heart, blood vessels, kidneys, eyes and nerves.

Damage to the small blood vessels and nerves

Constant high blood-glucose levels can cause damage to the linings of small blood vessels and nerves. This is very common in people with diabetes and is the first sign of many diabetes problems. Damage to these vessels can cause: kidney disease, eye damage and nerve damage.

Damage to large or medium blood vessels

Damage to the vessel linings leads to thickened and blocked arteries (large blood vessels) and can result in:

- heart attack
- stroke
- slow healing of cuts and scratches on the feet
- high blood pressure
- problems with erections for men
- pain in lower legs.

Heart

The risk of heart disease is increased for people who have diabetes. Heart disease occurs when the arteries supplying blood to the muscles of the heart become narrowed by deposits of cholesterol and damaged by poor diabetes control. If the narrowing decreases the blood supply to the heart too much, the heart muscle can be damaged. If vessels become blocked a heart attack can occur.

High blood pressure, high blood fats (cholesterol and triglyceride) and cigarette smoking also increase the risk of heart disease.

Report any chest pain or breathlessness to your doctor immediately.

Kidneys

Kidney disease is more common in people with diabetes. The kidneys filter waste products from the blood and get rid of them in the urine. The presence in the urine of small amounts of protein (micro albuminuria) could indicate that the filtering system has been damaged. Kidney function is monitored by your doctor testing your urine and blood.

Keeping blood glucose and blood pressure normal will reduce the risk of kidney damage.

Eyes

Diabetes can affect your eyes in different ways. In most cases the effects are temporary or can be helped by improving diabetes control. In some cases, however, the damage may cause permanent changes in your eyesight.

Diabetes can cause blurred vision. This can be due to raised blood-glucose levels altering the balance of fluid in the lens of the eye. Controlling blood-glucose levels can help prevent this change.

Eye problems can be prevented or delayed by controlling diabetes and blood pressure, avoiding smoking and having regular eye checks by your ophthalmologist or optometrist.

It is recommended that all people with diabetes have a complete eye examination at diagnosis and then regularly (at the interval advised by your healthcare team) throughout their lives. You should contact your doctor if you have any of the following symptoms:

- blurred vision that lasts longer than a day or so
- sudden loss of vision in either eye
- black spots, lines or flashing lights in your field of vision.

Cataracts: A cataract is the clouding of the normally clear lens of the eye. Cataracts commonly occur in older age. In people with diabetes, however, high blood glucose may speed up the development of cataracts. Blurred and dimmed vision are the first symptoms of a cataract. Cataracts can be removed and artificial lenses inserted.

Eye damage: The retina is the light-sensing tissue at the back of the eye. Damage to the retina (retinopathy) is caused by changes in the tiny vessels that supply the retina with blood. Regular checks with your ophthalmologist or optometrist are the best way to discover changes before your eyesight is affected and before the problem becomes harder to treat. The most effective treatment for retina damage is with lasers, which use a bright, powerful beam of light to treat the affected areas.

Infections
People with diabetes have an increased risk of infection, especially if blood-glucose levels are high or if blood vessels or nerves are damaged.

- *Skin*: Boils may occur and minor wounds may become infected.
- *Thrush*: Infections in the genital areas often caused by a fungus or 'yeast'. The vagina or the tip of the penis are most likely to be infected. Symptoms can be very annoying: irritation or redness and unpleasant discharge or odour.
- *Urine*: Infection may make you pass urine more often and experience a burning pain when passing urine and aching in the lower back or stomach. Drinking lots of water and taking medications to make the urine alkaline may reduce the symptoms.
- *Feet*: Small cuts or tinea between the toes may become infected.

Report any redness, swelling or increased temperature to your doctor, podiatrist or diabetes nurse.

If you have any of these symptoms, report them to your doctor immediately. Infections can be treated with antibiotics by mouth, injection or local application. However, treatment may not be effective until diabetes control has improved.

Nerve fibres

Damage to nerves is thought to be directly related to poor diabetes control. The nerves control muscles, carry messages to the brain and control functions such as digestion and blood pressure. Diabetes can cause changes in these nerves and the functions they control.

You may experience the following symptoms if your nerves are damaged — tell your doctor if you experience any of them:

- numbness and tingling in the hands or feet
- burning pains in the feet and legs
- erection problems
- dizziness
- loss of control or difficulty in passing urine
- indigestion
- alternating constipation and diarrhoea.

Feet and legs

Leg and foot problems in people with diabetes can be caused by damage to the blood vessels and nerves.

If the blood supply is reduced, you may experience pain in one or both of the calf muscles during and after exercise.

Cuts and scratches on your feet may heal slowly and, if not treated, become infected and form ulcers. In turn, if not treated quickly and effectively, ulcers may lead to the loss of all or part of the limb.

Diabetes can also dull the sensitivity of nerves. You might not feel the damage caused by tight shoes or the pressure of walking — if such damage is ignored, the foot can enlarge and become infected.

Proper foot care and footwear, along with regular visits to your doctor or podiatrist, can prevent leg and foot problems.

Illness and diabetes

Hyperglycaemia, or high blood glucose, often occurs when you are sick because illness and stress make the body's insulin work less effectively. With certain illnesses you may need to get to hospital to stabilise your diabetes.

Insulin injections may temporarily lower blood-glucose levels.

CHAPTER 2

LIVING WELL WITH DIABETES

Food, activity and relaxation are lifestyle issues that affect everyone for better or for worse. This is especially true if you have diabetes. Whether you have type 1 or type 2, it is important to follow a more healthy lifestyle.

Human beings are primarily hunter-gatherers. By necessity, we survived originally by catching and eating wild animals and fish for their lean meat, collecting fresh fruit, nuts and vegetables and gathering and cooking grains. Over millennia, our bodies gradually adapted to the high activity of hunting and gathering required to procure food, and to the low-fat, low-sugar dietary characteristics of the food itself.

We have come a long way since the Stone Age. Now, most of us in Western countries have lives of affluence. However, the way we are living does not suit our bodies. In the last half-century or so our lifestyle has changed dramatically but our bodies have not. Nature takes much longer to adapt to changes and many generations to evolve fully.

Our current lifestyle generally is characterised by less activity — no seeking and capturing prey or manually tilling, cultivating and harvesting vegetables and grains. Cars, buses, escalators and supermarkets provide for us now.

Much of our food is derived from intensively fed animals reared in confined spaces, or refined grains, or fried and sweet foods — all of which contain more fats and sugars than we are able to process. Bart Simpson's dad may like to sit watching TV, with a beer and chips, but he may not like the effects on his caveman body.

The same applies to all of us, and is especially true if you have diabetes. Whether you have type 1 or type 2 diabetes it is very important for you to follow a more healthy lifestyle to minimise the effects of our new affluence. This can be done by improving your diet and taking gentle exercise.

A healthy lifestyle

Remember, healthy food and exercise are two very important lifestyle issues.

Improving your diet

- *Watch your waist*: Excess fat is not healthy. The less extra fat your body has, the better it can function. Stay trim, taut and terrific.
- *Eat less fat*: Fat contains lots of energy, much of which you are probably unable to use. Any excessive fat may block your blood vessels impeding vital flow, so it is especially important to avoid trans fat and saturated fat.
- *Eat complex carbohydrate*: Fruit, vegetables and cereals all have complex carbohydrate and only small amounts of the sugars that increase blood-glucose levels.
- *Spread your complex carbohydrate*: Eating small quantities of food throughout the day spreads the load and gives a smooth, steady supply of glucose.

Exercise

- *Take 30*: Thirty minutes of moderate activity a day has been shown to help insulin to work and to help your blood vessels to stay healthy.

Stress and the city hunter

For the human animal, a 'stress' situation occurs when danger threatens. We have two options: either fight or take flight. Our bodies get ready: our breathing deepens to provide more oxygen, our heart speeds up to pump more blood to the muscles, our muscles tense in preparation to strike or run — and our stores of glucose are released and re-distributed to ensure that additional energy is available as required.

A stress situation such as this is fine for the Stone Age human whose body was honed for such an event, but it is bad news for the modern city dweller with diabetes — the last thing you want is for the glucose stored in your body to be freely released. It shouldn't surprise you that stress can push up your blood glucose. Your body has trouble enough keeping glucose stored in the right place without stress pushing it out again. Reflect on a stressful situation that you have been involved in: maybe narrowly missing having an accident in a car or being startled by someone when you thought you were alone. Your heart raced and you were probably left with a sick unsteady feeling.

Stress makes controlling blood glucose more difficult. Modern society cultivates stress — there are more people around, more intensive demands on our lifestyle, bad drivers, traffic lights, and so on. There's enough to cope with already without the additional stress of diabetes.

Unfortunately you cannot avoid all the stresses of everyday life. But you can reduce stress and help your body deal with it when it occurs.

There are lots of ways of helping your body deal with stress:

- *Get out of that chair!* Regular activity is one way to reduce stress and it helps to keep your weight and blood vessels healthy as well.
- *Take time out*: Make time for you to be yourself. Enjoy activities and hobbies that relax you. Ensure that you allocate some 'quality time' to yourself.
- *Join in a community activity*: Check your local community centre for relaxation, fitness and exercise programs. Group activity enhances wellbeing and reduces the isolation of stress.
- *Take up tai chi*: The mental harmony and gentle movements of tai chi are an ideal stressbuster, enabling the body to adjust and balance itself naturally.

Drinkwise

Alcohol 'drinkwise' equals 'two for men and women one'.

This slogan refers to standard drinks that contain 10 grams of alcohol — 300 millilitres of beer or 100 millilitres of wine. In moderation — two drinks for men and one drink for women — alcohol is pleasant, sociable and safe as long as you don't drink on an empty stomach. However, alcohol can cause three special problems in people with diabetes:

1. *Weight gain*: Alcohol has lots of energy you may not need if you are trying to control your weight.
2. *Loss of judgement*: The relaxed feeling may lead you to make some decisions about food or medication that you regret later.
3. *Low blood glucose*: Just as stress releases glucose stores, alcohol can block the release and cause low blood glucose.

Generally, it is better to drink alcohol with food. There are many suitable choices, but some have lots of sugar and are best avoided. The better choices are dry wines, such as riesling, dry reds, brut champagnes and dry sherry, and spirits such as whisky, brandy, gin, rum, vodka and dry vermouth — but in moderation. Always choose a 'diet' mixer.

Golden guidelines

1. Watch your waist.
2. Eat less fat.
3. Eat complex carbohydrate.
4. Spread your complex carbohydrate.
5. Take regular exercise.
6. Take time out.
7. Quit smoking for life.
8. Drinkwise: two drinks for men, one for women.

Golden guidelines are all very well, but what should you actually do? Here are some practical things you need to know.

1. Watch your waist

Excess fat is not healthy. How fat are you? Should you lose weight? Your waist will tell you: the most dangerous fat is stored in your tummy. Doctors have studied fats in the body by tracing them with radioactive isotopes and have found that the fats in the tummy tend to block your heart and arteries; fat in the hip and chest won't harm you. Below is a guide, although it varies according to your height and body shape.

	Healthy waist	Overweight waist	Very overweight waist
For men	under 94 cm	94–102 cm	over 102 cm
For women	under 80 cm	80–88 cm	over 88 cm

See your doctor, diabetes nurse or dietitian for expert advice if you do need to lose weight around your waist area.

2. Eat less fat

Are you eating fatty foods? Should you change your eating and cooking habits? Keep a food diary and write down everything you eat for one week. (No cheating!)

Now check for fatty foods listed in the checklist below. Consider trying the alternative food choices. Make the healthy choice and stop buying and cooking fatty foods. That way you, your family and your friends will all be better off.

✗ Avoid or limit — high in fat	✓ Suitable alternatives
✗ *Oily dressings:* mayonnaise, cream sauces, fatty gravies, sour cream	✓ *Low-joule (low-calorie) dressings:* vinegar, lemon juice, low-joule gravy, plain unsweetened yoghurt
✗ *Fat in meat:* chicken skin, fatty meats, sausages, fritz, bacon, salami, deep-fried foods, pies, pasties	✓ *Reduced fat:* skinless chicken, lean cuts of meat, foods cooked without fat or with minimal amount of vegetable oil
✗ *Snack foods:* nuts, crisps, corn chips	✓ *Fresh fruit and vegetables:* crisp, raw vegies, fruit and plain popcorn
✗ *Fats:* large amounts of margarine, butter, oil, cream, peanut butter, dripping, lard, ghee	✓ *Limit fat:* 3–6 teaspoons per day, preferably polyunsaturated margarine or oil

3. Eat complex carbohydrate *and*

4. Spread your complex carbohydrate

Check your food diary. Do you eat a lot of sugar or sugary foods? See the sugar checklist below and consider alternatives.

Do you have complex starchy food each time you eat? A regular, moderate intake of unrefined carbohydrates, spread over at least three meals a day, helps reduce fluctuation in blood-glucose levels over the day. The more spread out the carbohydrate intake the better — three small meals with some inbetween-meal snacks is often the best.

Because the recommended diet is low in fat, the carbohydrate content will be relatively high. It is important that it is the right type of carbohydrate — relatively unrefined and high in fibre, which is slowly absorbed. Particularly good choices include beans, lentils, oats, pasta and fresh fruit. And instead of having foods that contain lots of sugar, eat more fresh fruit and vegetables.

✗ Avoid or limit — high in sugar	✓ Suitable alternatives
✗ Sugar, honey	✓ *Artificial sweetener:* tablet or liquid
✗ *Spreads:* jam, marmalade, syrups, Nutella	✓ *Low-joule (low-calorie) spreads:* jam, marmalade, Promite, Vegemite, meat or fish paste
✗ *Sweet drinks:* cordial, soft drink, flavoured mineral water, tonic water, fruit juice drinks, flavoured milk, milkshakes, sweet wine, sherry, port, liqueurs, ordinary beer	✓ *Low-joule (low-calorie) drinks:* cordial, soft drink, plain mineral water, soda water, pure fruit juice (limit 1 small glass/day), coffee, tea, herb teas, dry wine, spirits, low alcohol beer (1–2 drinks/day).
✗ *Confectionary:* lollies, cough lollies, chocolate (ordinary, diabetic, carob), muesli/health bars.	✓ *Healthy substitutes:* crackers, crispbreads, wheat-meal
✗ Sweet biscuits and cakes, sweet pastries, doughnuts	✓ *Low-joule desserts:* jelly, fresh or tinned/stewed fruit without sugar, custard/junket made with liquid sweetener, plain or diet-lite yoghurt.
✗ Sweet cereals such as some mueslis, Nutrigrain, Cocopops, Honeysmacks.	✓ *Other cereals:* porridge, Weetbix, Allbran, ready wheats

5. Take regular exercise

Consider some simple ways of increasing your physical activity:

- Use stairs instead of lifts.
- Perform housework and shopping at a brisk pace.
- Go walking during your lunch break — in fact, walk whenever you can.
- Create an excuse to be active — moving around is better than sitting around. Walk to the shops, don't drive. Get a dog, and take it for a daily walk. Go to the park and throw a ball around with your kids. Take swimming lessons. Join a gym.

Add Tai Chi for Diabetes to your life. The great thing about the Tai Chi for Diabetes program is that almost anyone can do it. Tai chi differs from many other exercises popular in Western countries — for example, it's slow, which may be a challenge for some because we're used to a fast-pace life. But once you get used to tai chi's calming tempo, you'll find it surprisingly enjoyable. In nature, slow complements fast. After studying tai chi for three months, most people become interested in it and enjoy practicing it for years.

Tai Chi for Diabetes can be adapted to your own specific needs. You can take it simply as a gentle and pleasant exercise. Adapting the philosophical understanding of nature and tai chi as a way of life helps you become more relaxed and tranquil — and, in time, this can help you cope better with your condition. You can incorporate any of the tai chi principles — such as good posture, maintaining good mental and physical balance — into your daily routine to help you live better with diabetes (see chapter 3, The Healing Power of Tai Chi).

6. Take time out

Put aside some part of the day that you can call your own and do something you want to do. Decide on a time — morning tea, lunch, after the shopping, after work — and stick to it. Go and sit in a café by yourself and read a book or magazine for thirty minutes. Spend the afternoon at the movies. Turn off your mobile and go to the beach.

Find out more about relaxation. Go to the council, the library, or ask your doctor or healthcare team.

7. Quit smoking for life

Make the decision. If you are a heavy smoker or have had trouble giving up before, you may need help. Talk to your healthcare team. Enquire about self-help groups at your council or community health centre.

Set the date for quitting. Persuade your partner to stop too. Write the date down and tell your friends. Put up notices and ask friends and family to remind you and encourage you each week. Find a substitute, an activity such as a sport or tai chi, something you like which you can become 'addicted' to — but something that is good for you. Think about situations when you will be tempted to smoke and work out how you will deal with them or avoid them for a while. Don't worry if you make a few mistakes — keep trying. You can do it.

Ring the Quitline anytime you need support.

8. Drinkwise: two for men, one for women

As with smoking, make the decision to stick to the healthy limit. Work out the times you will be tempted to drink alcohol and how you will deal with the situation (or avoid it for a while).

> DON'T WORRY IF YOU MAKE A FEW
> MISTAKES — KEEP AT IT.

Managing your condition

Managing your diabetes well is the key to a more fulfilled and happier life. Take some time to work out what your objectives in your life are, what makes you happy and fulfilled. It may be to be a useful member of your family, to do well at your work, to pursue the things you enjoy or to gain respect and recognition. Almost anything that makes you feel more fulfilled, fitter, stronger, healthier and happier will be enhanced if you manage your diabetes well. And it will be hindered if your diabetes is poorly controlled.

A simple way to approach managing your condition is to work out a plan based on your objectives and identify how diabetes may limit these objectives. Make it practical and workable for you — for example, if you have problems losing weight, it is unlikely you are going to reach your perfect body weight overnight; but if you plan to lose 1 to 2 kilograms per month, it is more manageable (and the weight is more likely to stay off).

Once you've made your plan, stick to it. Your diabetes care team may be able to help you.

When it comes to the crunch, though, you are the one who has to take care of your condition and develop a way to manage it effectively. You will get back what you put in.

People often feel the way to manage a condition is to go and see the doctor, get a pill prescribed, take the pill and be fixed. But some medical conditions are much more complicated, especially diabetes. Most health professionals encourage self-management of conditions by patients — studies show that people with chronic conditions such as arthritis and diabetes do better with self-management.

That doesn't mean you need to become a doctor to manage your condition. It means that you manage your own condition in conjunction with your health professionals and diabetes team. The team members may include: your family doctor, your diabetes specialist, your heart specialist (if appropriate), diabetes educators, podiatrist, dietician, nurse, family members, your friends, tai chi teacher and exercise and fitness teachers. They are your consultants and assistants and you are the manager who learns as much as you can about how best to take their advice and apply it to your life.

Your doctor, for example, would advise you to eat less fat and more complex carbohydrates. If your long-term goal is to be healthier and fitter and do a good job at your workplace, or be helpful to your family, then resist the temptation for the temporary gratification from eating a piece of cake and follow your doctor's advice. It is good advice, of course. In the long run you will enjoy your life more because you are healthier and are able to handle all aspects of your life better. And if you ignore the advice and have uncontrolled diabetes, it is much more likely that you will get complications, such as heart attack or stroke. Certainly you are less likely to reach your goal, and you may become a burden to your family.

Tablets

Diabetes tablets lower blood-glucose levels and are used by people whose bodies make insulin (if insulin levels are too low, insulin injections are required). The tablets are not insulin, which would not work if taken by mouth because they would be broken down in the stomach. Tablets work best when your weight is controlled by healthy eating and activity.

There are five types of tablets commonly used: metformin, sulphonylureas, glitazones, glitinides and acarbose (the last three are not often used). Although the action of most diabetes tablets is not fully understood, they work in two main ways: by reducing the body's resistance to insulin or by increasing the amount of insulin produced.

- *Metformin* reduces insulin resistance and helps the body respond to insulin. It also helps with weight loss in some people.
- *Sulphonylureas* stimulate the pancreas to make more insulin.

- The *glitazones*, like metformin, reduce insulin resistance and help the body respond to insulin.
- The *glitinides* are like short-acting sulphonylureas and briefly increase insulin levels at meal times.
- *Acarbose* slows the absorption of carbohydrate (starchy) foods.

A doctor will prescribe a specific medication based on your general health and how much your blood-glucose levels need to be lowered. Your eating habits, weight and any possible side effects of the medication will also determine the choice of drug.

Side effects

Oral diabetes medications may cause the following side effects in some people. Your doctor should explain these to you when prescribing medication. Be sure to check with your doctor if you suspect any side effects from your medication.

- *Metformin*: flatulence and/or diarrhoea, nausea and/or loss of appetite.
- *Sulphonylureas*: hypoglycaemia (low blood glucose) if meals are missed or activity increased (see page 4), weight gain.
- *Glitazones*: weight gain, fluid accumulation.
- *Glitinides*: hypoglycaemia and weight gain (less likely than with sulphonylureas).
- *Acarbose*: flatulence and/or diarrhoea.

Advice on taking tablets

If you are taking diabetes tablets, note the following important points:

- If possible take tablets as prescribed regarding their timing and in relation to meals and at the same time each day.
- Try not to miss or delay meals.
- Some other medications can react with diabetes tablets — for

example, medications for blood pressure, arthritis and asthma. Discuss this with your doctor or pharmacist.

- Do not take more or less tablets than your doctor prescribes.
- Consult your doctor if you need to stop your tablets for any reason.
- Know the name and dose of your tablets (keep a note of these details somewhere handy).
- Store tablets in their airtight containers away from direct sunlight.
- Most diabetes tablets are not suitable for pregnant women; consult your doctor if you suspect you are pregnant.
- Consult your doctor or pharmacist if you have any questions about your diabetes tablets or any other medication.

Insulin

There are times when people with type 2 diabetes might need insulin: when blood-glucose levels are not controlled by healthy lifestyle and diabetes tablets and, temporarily, to control blood glucose in special situations such as surgery and pregnancy.

If you need insulin injections, your doctor and diabetes nurse will teach you how to purchase, mix and inject insulin. These days injections are much easier because of insulin pens: these are like a fountain pen with a needle and cartridge of insulin instead of a nib and cartridge of ink. These pens are easier to carry and use than injections.

Further information on the action and use of insulin can also be provided by diabetes organisations (see Resources, page 174).

Beyond blood glucose

Blood-glucose control may not be the only priority. Type 2 diabetes increases the risk of heart attacks and strokes (see page 9) and is often associated with other risk factors for blood-vessel damage. High pressure in the arteries damages blood vessels and the heart. High cholesterol settles in the arteries and could block them — if the damage causes a clot, a heart attack or stroke occurs. You need to learn your ABCs again. Getting to, and staying at, your targets protects you against heart attacks and strokes. Ask your doctor what your 'numbers' are? Are you on target? If not, talk to your doctor about how you might get there.

Keeping track of glucose levels

It is important to keep track of your diabetes. This requires regularly checking the amount of glucose in your blood. Your doctor can measure your blood glucose during a visit to the surgery, and you can test and record your levels at home. This enables you to keep a day-to-day check on how you are controlling your diabetes.

What to aim for

Glucose levels go up and down throughout the day. Blood-glucose levels are usually lower before meals and after exercise. Higher levels occur after meals and when you are under stress. Successful diabetes management requires you to maintain a careful balance between your food, activity and diabetes medication.

Checking your diabetes

Blood glucose monitoring

Today many people measure blood-glucose levels with a simple and accurate blood test which can be done at home.

Such blood tests require only a single drop of blood, which you can obtain by pricking your finger. The blood is placed on a test strip and the result can be read on a meter or with a colour chart. This allows you to check your blood-glucose levels at any time. Discuss with your doctor the best times to test.

BLOOD GLUCOSE LEVEL

There are two measurement systems for measuring blood glucose levels: the 'world standard' of mmol/L and the US system of mg/dL. One mmol/L is one millimole of glucose per litre of blood and one mg/dL is one milligram of glucose per decilitre of blood. The simple way to convert is to multiply or divide by 18.

Below are some important readings to keep in mind, a blood glucose level of 5 mmol/L is equivalent to about one-sixth of a teaspoon of glucose per litre of blood.

mmol/L	mg/dL	Fingertip Blood Sample Level
2	36	dangerously low
3	54	too low
4	70	low but still within normal limit
8	144	maximum for non-diabetes
15	270	dangerously high

Urine testing

The presence of glucose in the urine may indicate that there is too much glucose in the blood. When glucose levels get too high in the blood, the kidneys are unable to remove the excess glucose, which spills out into the urine. The level at which this occurs is called the renal threshold. Urine testing can provide an indication of blood-glucose levels if the renal threshold has been reached. Urine testing is only recommended when blood-glucose testing is not possible.

The A1c

Your doctor or nurse may do this test to assess your blood-glucose control over several months. Also known as glycosylated haemoglobin

(HbA1c), the test measures the amount of glucose attached to haemoglobin during the life span of red cells.

Glucose in the blood attaches to red blood cells; the part of the cell that carries oxygen is called haemoglobin and has a life span of about 120 days. If blood-glucose levels are high, then a greater amount of glucose attaches to the haemoglobin. This measurement is the average of 'highs' and 'lows' of blood-glucose levels over the past few months.

Out of balance

The aim of diabetes treatment is to keep blood-glucose levels as close to normal range as possible. If you have diabetes, your body is no longer able to maintain this control. You will need to balance your food, activity, lifestyle and medication.

High glucose

High blood-glucose levels (hyperglycaemia) can occur in any person with diabetes.

Very high blood-glucose levels (above 15 mmol/L or 270 mg/dL) can make you feel tired and unwell. You may pass urine more often than usual, which will make you thirsty. Your vision may become blurred (see page 3).

High blood-glucose levels can occur if you:

- eat too much sugary or starchy food at one time
- consume too many drinks high in sugar
- are inactive, causing your insulin or tablets to work less efficiently
- are overweight
- have an illness or infection
- experience emotional stress (for example, family conflict)
- miss your dose of tablets or insulin, or if the dose is too low
- take certain medications such as prednisolone (discuss this further with your doctor or pharmacist).

Low glucose

If your blood-glucose levels are very low (under 3 mmol/L or 54 mg/dL), a condition called hypoglycaemia results. Low blood-glucose levels (hypoglycaemia) can only occur in people taking some diabetes tablets or insulin.

You may feel shaky, nervous and very weak. You may sweat, feel hungry and have a headache. If hypoglycaemia is not treated, your speech may become slurred and you will appear confused, irritable and drowsy. Severe hypoglycaemia can cause loss of consciousness.

A person with hypoglycaemia who is conscious should eat or drink something containing sugar, such as sweetened orange juice, regular lemonade or jelly beans — it will require five or six jelly beans to avert a hypoglycaemic attach — or you can get a glucose pack from your pharmacy just for this purpose. Follow this with some long-acting carbohydrate food, such as a wholemeal sandwich or a piece of fruit.

If the person is unconscious, do not try to give them fluids or food. They will require an injection (of glucagon) to raise their blood-glucose level. Call an ambulance or take them to hospital immediately.

In order to prevent future occurrence, it is important to identify what caused the hypoglycaemia.

Low blood-glucose levels can occur if you:

- miss or delay meals or snacks
- are unwell and cannot eat properly
- do strenuous activities without eating extra carbohydrate
- drink too much alcohol
- do not take your correct dose of tablets (or insulin), or if the dose is too high
- have had significant weight loss.

PRECAUTIONS

Always wear identification so health professionals can find out your medical condition and medications if you are involved in an accident or have a serious illness and are unconscious or unable to speak.

High glucose

- When your blood-glucose levels are high, check your diet, exercise and medication to see if you can find a cause.
- Don't omit or reduce your tablet/insulin dose without the advice of your doctor.
- If you have high blood-glucose levels above 15 mmol/L as defined by your healthcare team, contact your doctor or diabetes nurse.

Low glucose

- If you take tablets or insulin, you should always carry sweets, such as jelly beans, and eat them at the first sign of a 'hypo'. Remember that you will need to eat five or six jelly beans to avert a hypoglycaemic attack.
- The effect of hypoglycaemia should be explained to relatives, friends and work mates, so they will know how to help you.

- If you have frequent occurrences of hypoglycaemia, you should contact your doctor or diabetes nurse.

Foot care

People with diabetes have a lower resistance to infection, and often have poorer circulation, particularly to the feet. Any minor injury can lead to serious infection and sometimes amputation. So it is important to take care of your feet.

- Inspect your feet daily.
- Wash your feet daily and carefully 'pat' them dry.
- Take care to dry between your toes.

Toe nails

- Wash your feet before cutting nails.
- Always cut your nails straight across and use an emery board to gently round the edges.
- Be careful not to cut the skin.
- Don't cut your nails shorter than the top of your toe.
- If your toes are ingrown, very thick or tend to split, consult a podiatrist.
- If your eyesight is impaired, have a family member inspect your feet daily and trim your nails when required.

Footwear

- Wear shoes (preferably leather) that cover your feet and provide airholes for ventilation.
- Never wear tight-fitting shoes.
- Wear cotton or wool-mix socks.
- Make sure all socks are roomy and do not restrict movement.
- Do not wear knee-high stockings or garters because they might restrict your circulation.

Avoid damage
- Don't go barefoot if the blood vessels or nerves to your feet are damaged, or if you are somewhere that is stony or where you are likely to cut your feet.
- Do not use electric blankets or hot water bottles.
- Do not sit too close to heaters.

Treating minor foot problems
- If you notice dry or rough skin, gently rub wet feet with a pumice stone. At night rub in a moisturising cream.
- If the skin is very dry, use an oil-based cream such as lanolin for two to three days until skin has improved.
- Treat cuts and abrasions immediately: wash your feet in soap and water then dry carefully. If the cut is unclean, wash feet in a very mild disinfectant and apply a mild antiseptic to the injured area. Consult your doctor or podiatrist if the injury doesn't improve in 24 hours.

Illness and diabetes

Hyperglycaemia often occurs when you are sick because illness and stress make the body's insulin work less effectively. With certain illnesses, you may need to go to hospital to stabilise your diabetes.

Insulin injections may temporarily lower blood-glucose levels. During illness you should:

- never reduce or stop taking your dose of tablets or insulin without consulting your doctor
- test your blood glucose every two to four hours, especially if you are on insulin
- if you are on insulin, test your urine for ketones
- if you are nauseated and unable to eat, increase your fluid intake and drink regular lemonade, sweetened fruit juices or sugared water (one-quarter to one glass half-hourly); check with your doctor if it

lasts for more than twelve hours and, likewise, if you cannot drink, consult your doctor

- rest, do not exercise
- consult your doctor if vomiting occurs, the illness persists or your diabetes remains unstable.

Oral hygiene

Oral hygiene is very important for people with diabetes because you are more likely to develop infection. Visit your dentist regularly to ensure any existing problems are treated immediately and to learn how to take care of your mouth, gums and teeth. Tell your dentist that you have diabetes.

Your dentist or dental hygienist can give you advice on the correct techniques of mouth, gum and teeth care.

If you require tooth extraction or a general anaesthetic for any dental work, you or your dentist may need to contact your doctor or diabetes specialist for advice. Preparation for an anaesthetic of any type may involve alteration to your usual diabetes management.

Shared responsibilities

You can do a lot to improve your own treatment. The following points will help you.

Routine self-care

- Try to lose excess weight and not regain it.
- Learn about which healthy foods to choose and how to prepare them. Use available resources to develop a wide range of recipes.
- Develop a regular program of physical activities you enjoy and adhere to it — consider giving the Tai Chi for Diabetes program a try (see page 92).
- Ensure you always have enough medication.

- Monitor your blood-glucose and/or urine levels regularly.
- Wash and inspect your feet daily.
- Visit your doctor regularly.
- Visit your dentist regularly.

Year-to-year self-care

- Get a MedicAlert bracelet.
- Join an ambulance fund.
- Join your national diabetes organisation and services schemes (see Resources, page 174).
- Get involved in a local support, walking or cookery group.
- Check whether you need to update your tetanus toxoid status (you need an injection at age fifty).
- Consider getting vaccinated against flu and pneumonia — discuss this with your doctor.
- Arrange regular appointments with an ophthalmologist or an optometrist (at the recommended intervals) and a podiatrist.

Visit your doctor

Remember you are the most important member of your healthcare team. Discuss the management of your diabetes with your healthcare team.

Make an appointment at the interval advised by your doctor (usually every three to six months) to check:

- weight
- diabetes management — including your blood-glucose records and A1c
- medications
- injection site (if you are on insulin)
- eyes: visual sharpness
- kidney function (urine and blood tests)
- feet.

Your doctor may also refer you to other specialist health professionals such as your ophthalmologist.

Smoking

Smoking is unhealthy for everyone. But it is particularly dangerous for people with diabetes because it can lead to heart disease and circulation problems. Smoking also reduces your fitness. If you are a smoker and are having trouble quitting, talk to your doctor and contact Quitline (see Resources, page 174).

Sex and contraception

Sex, like any other activity, requires energy. If you are being treated with insulin, you may need to eat extra food beforehand to avoid hypoglycaemia.

Long-standing diabetes in a man can occasionally cause erectile problems. If problems occur, treatment may help. Any sexual problems or worries can be discussed with your doctor or diabetes nurse.

There is no perfect form of contraception. Ask your doctor or family planning clinic about the best method of contraception for you. Plan pregnancies so your diabetes is controlled, which will avoid problems for both you and your child.

Employment

For most people with type 2 diabetes, diabetes has no effect on their work. Your abilities are as good as before you developed diabetes — perhaps even better if you start living a more healthy lifestyle.

However, there are some occupations that are unsuitable for people with diabetes if they are at risk of becoming unconscious because of low glucose levels or of not coping because of high glucose levels. These include occupations where your safety or the safety of others may be put at risk — for example, driving public transport, using dangerous machinery or where heights are involved.

In most situations, this only applies to people treated with tablets (although some tablets don't cause hypoglycemia — your doctor can advise you on this) or insulin, which can cause hypoglycaemia.

If your job involves shift work, discuss any necessary adjustments to your routine with your doctor, dietitian or diabetes nurse.

If you are on tablets or insulin that can cause hypoglycaemia (see page 4), it is also important to make sure someone you work with is aware you have diabetes and understands the symptoms and treatment for hypoglycaemia.

Travel

Travel can and should be fun, but a few precautions need to be taken to avoid problems.

If you are not on insulin, you should not have any problems in continuing your normal routine. However, expect and be prepared for:

- changes in temperature
- a change in activity
- time zone changes
- different food
- sightseeing tours
- misplaced luggage — take some medication in your hand luggage
- unexpected delays.

If you are travelling by car:

- have regular meals and snacks at the usual times
- carry extra food and drink in case of delays
- stop for short breaks and take the time for a walk
- wear or carry identification

- carry quick-acting carbohydrates, such as sweets or soft drinks, and long-acting carbohydrates, such as dry biscuits and fruit (see pages 36 for further information)
- if you take insulin or tablets that cause hypoglycaemia (see pages 30–31), watch out for its onset and treat it immediately; move into the back seat while you are recovering so the police can see you are not driving 'under the influence of a drug that could affect your judgement'.

If you are travelling by bus, train or plane, follow the above points. In addition:

- alert the attendant about your need for meals
- be as active as possible
- carry tablets and testing equipment in your hand luggage; also keep one set of supplies in separate luggage.

If you are travelling overseas, you may need to change your tablets and lifestyle routines. Talk to your healthcare. If on insulin, you should discuss your travel arrangements with your doctor or diabetes nurse:

- check your blood glucose more than usual while travelling
- always take out medical insurance
- check the strength of any insulin you are prescribed when travelling
- check what documents you need to take with you.

Medicines and supplies

In some countries, there are national or state schemes where you can obtain the cheapest blood- and urine-testing strips and other supplies. Check with your local diabetes organisation.

A prescription is required to purchase all diabetes medications. Urine and blood-glucose monitoring strips can also be provided through the pharmacies, with or without prescriptions.

Blood-glucose meters can be bought from diabetes organisations, some hospital clinics and pharmacies. Make sure you understand how to use and maintain the meter and what you are to do if the blood-glucose values are too high or too low. See Resources, page 174.

Guidelines for non-prescription medicines

When purchasing non-prescription medicines:

- read labels carefully: check ingredients, warnings and precautions — and if you are worried about the warnings or precautions, discuss your concerns with your doctor or pharmacist
- choose tablets or capsules rather than liquid medicines, which are more likely to contain alcohol and/or sugar
- low-dose aspirin (for example, 100 mg/day) is very likely to affect diabetes tablets; high-dose aspirin (4000 mg/day) can.

Insurance, driving and legal obligations

Travel insurance

Some insurance companies do not provide overseas travel insurance for people with a pre-existing, long-term illness such as diabetes. If you are planning to travel overseas you could discuss the best options for travel insurance with your local diabetes organisation or your diabetes nurse.

Life insurance or superannuation

Inform your insurance company that you have diabetes. In some situations premiums may be adjusted. An insurance broker can assist you if your require further information.

Motor vehicle licences

If you take diabetes tablets, you may be required to notify the motor vehicle registrar and your car insurance company; if you use insulin, you must notify both.

It is an offence to drive without such notification and you may incur a heavy penalty. In addition, your insurance cover may be invalidated if you don't notify your insurance company. Check requirements with the insurance company and motor vehicle registrar.

Stress and diabetes

Most people struggle with the diagnosis of diabetes. Adjusting to new routines of eating, medication use and concerns over health can all be sources of stress.

Managing stress is important for everyone, but particularly for those with diabetes — stress can make it much harder for you to self-manage the condition.

You need to be aware of your stress levels, the way you respond and the sources of the stress. Some forms of short-term stress are useful because they motivate you to face challenges and to improve performance. However, other forms, such as long-term stress, can affect your ability to cope and your emotional and physical well being.

Stress: what can you do?

Awareness

Be aware of your stress levels. It is important to notice, for example, when you are tense, worried, irritable or having trouble concentrating. Awareness allows you to take early action to deal with the stress.

Problem-solving

Is the source of stress related to your living with diabetes? Can your health professional assist you in problem-solving and making informed decisions about your diabetes? Problem-solving can be a useful step in dealing with other sources of stress.

Whose problem is it?

Sometimes we take on other people's problems and the associated stress. It is always important to ask yourself 'Whose problem is this?' and to recognise that not all problems are yours to solve.

Resolution of problems

Not all problems have immediate solutions. In such situations, the best option is just to accept this. Ask yourself, 'Can I do anything about this right now?' If the answer is 'yes', do it; if the answer is 'no', accept this and do other things to alleviate your stress.

Thought patterns

If you consistently have negative thoughts about yourself that make it difficult for you to cope with stress consider obtaining professional help to recognise and change these patterns.

Managing time

Learn to set priorities for the demands on your time. Set goals that are achievable and have realistic expectations of the time it will take to achieve these. Remember to recognise and reward yourself as you take the steps towards your goals.

Assertiveness

Learn to say 'no' in the nicest possible way when you feel overloaded or simply do not want to do something. You cannot be all things to all people. If you fear the consequences of being assertive, take an assertiveness training course; ask your healthcare team for a recommendation.

Exercise

Regular exercise is recognised as one of the best ways to manage stress. Aim to include regular exercise, such as walking, bike riding, tai chi or fitness classes, into your weekly routine.

Short muscle relaxation exercises

Follow some or each of the exercises below. Do them in a sitting position and be careful not to over-tense your muscles — feel the tension and relax. (The Tai Chi for Diabetes program includes a short qigong exercise for relaxation, see page 96.)

- Stretch your fingers right out.
- Make a tight fist with your hand.
- Bend your hand from the wrist.
- Bend your arm from the elbow.
- Straighten and stretch your arm out.
- Stretch both arms out and push against an invisible barrier.
- Push your elbows into the back of your chair.
- Push your toes into the floor.
- Bend your feet up.
- Push your knees together tightly.
- Straighten both legs and push against an invisible wall.
- Clench your buttocks together.
- Press your abdomen into the back of the chair.
- Push your spine into the back of the chair.
- Shrug your shoulders towards your ears and drop them down slowly.
- Press your elbows to your sides and feel your chest muscles.
- Press your chin towards your chest gently.
- Push your tongue against the roof of your mouth.
- Wrinkle your nose.
- Screw up your eyes tightly.
- Tense everything — every muscle you can remember, and then relax.

If, after trying some of these exercises and the techniques mentioned above, you still feel stressed, contact your doctor, who may be able to put you in touch with a local group or with someone who has faced similar problems.

Breathing techniques

Focusing on your breathing is one way to manage acute stress. Use it when you get stressed at traffic lights or in a supermarket queue. Breathe in slowly to a count of three, hold your breath for a second and then breathe out slowly to a count of three. Aim for about ten breaths a minute. Note that this is not deep breathing but slow breathing. Or do the dan tian breathing method on page 107.

RELAXING WITH IMAGERY

Visualise a place where you are happy and content — this may be your own sitting room, a beach or a meadow by a river. Close your eyes and establish regular, gentle breathing. Visualise your scene. Using all your senses, slowly go through what you can see, what you can hear, what you can smell and what you can touch. Hold the image. When you want to stop, breathe deeply and slowly and count from one to three, reaching full alertness but maintaining a relaxed state.

The Tai Chi for Diabetes program

The mental harmony and gentle movements of tai chi make it an ideal 'stressbuster', enabling the body to adjust and balance itself naturally. Once you have become accustomed to its rhythm and feel, tai chi is enjoyable to do: it is natural for the body to have a balanced rhythm of fastness and slowness. With the Tai Chi for Diabetes program, most people can learn the basic set and qigong exercises within three months and may start gaining health benefits soon. If you're suffering from stress the benefits can be felt soon after you start.

Yoga and meditation

These can be very useful stress management techniques for some people, as can other forms of spiritual practice.

Remember

Stress managed well can build up your resilience. Aim to balance your work, health commitments, family, friends, exercise and relaxation. As you manage your stress, be willing to accept help from others and recognise and reward your own achievements.

If diabetes is the problem

Perhaps it would help to talk to people who understand what it's like to have the condition. Check out your local diabetes organisation.

Your healthcare team

When you are diagnosed with diabetes, as well as your family doctor you will need a team of health professionals who will monitor your condition and assist you in its management.

Diabetes nurse (also called diabetes nurse educator): Health professional (a registered nurse) who specialises in educating people about diabetes, including blood glucose/urine monitoring, administration of medications and lifestyle. Some have had special training and are *credentialled diabetes nurse educators* (CDE).

Dietitian: Provides dietary education, assessment and counselling regarding meal planning.

Endocrinologist: Medical specialist (physician) who treats people who have disorders of the endocrine glands, such as the pancreas.

Ophthalmologist: Medical specialist (physician) who treats the eye.

Optometrist: Measures errors in refraction of the eye's lens and prescribes glasses to correct the errors; is able to detect many eye conditions.

Orthopaedic surgeon: Surgical specialist (physician) who specialises in treating the musculoskeletal system.

Pharmacist: Prepares and dispenses medicines and provides advice on their use.

Physiotherapist: Uses physical measures (heat, cold, water, etc) to evaluate and treat disease and disability. Therapeutic exercises and training procedures are also used.

Podiatrist: Treats feet and gives advice on foot care and footwear.

Psychologist: Counsels people regarding the emotional aspects of illness.

Social worker: Counsels individuals and families regarding personal, family or marital problems and provides information about community resources.

Vascular surgeon: Surgical specialist (physician) who treats the blood vessels supplying body tissues.

Exercise leader: There are many levels of training in this field; a good exercise leader can guide you in the right and safe type of exercise.

Tai chi teacher: There are many forms of tai chi, and in most countries no standardised training for teachers. Be sure to find a teacher who understands your condition and is willing to be part of your healthcare team.

Working with your team

Before you start tai chi, be sure to discuss it with your doctor and diabetes health professionals. The amount and the extent of your exercise can affect your diabetes management, especially if you are on insulin or medication that may cause hypoglycaemia.

Describe the duration and the exertion level of your exercise to your healthcare team. We recommend you take this book with you. You can control the exertion level at any stage of your tai chi practice: as a general guide, the Tai Chi for Diabetes program is designed with very low physical exertion at the start, equivalent to slow walking. As you progress, however, it becomes comparable to normal walking. After you have learned the complete program, the exertion level is similar to that of brisk walking. You can control and adjust the level of exertion at any stage of the program.

You should report to your health professionals any changes in your physical/mental condition, including beneficial effects. As your condition improves, your healthcare team may need to adjust your medical treatment: for example, lowering the dosage of your medication.

It is an excellent idea to ask a friend, your family and support group to join you doing the tai chi program. This way, they would know how much exertion you have done, and all of you can enjoy something refreshingly different. Sometimes your supporting team might feel drained from caring for you — doing tai chi together will not only improve your condition (thus making their job easier), it will also energise them and improve their health. Tai Chi for Diabetes is suitable for almost anyone — it will provide many health benefits for people with or without diabetes.

Why tai chi for diabetes?

Exercising and being active are essential for good health — and even more so for diabetes management. It is important to find an exercise or activity that resonates with you so that you will keep to it. Tai chi, one of the most popular exercises in the world, appeals to people from all ages, backgrounds, and physical conditions. Almost anyone can take up tai chi and it does not require expensive equipment, much space or a lot of time. It is also intrinsically enjoyable — people enjoy the health benefits, serenity of mind and happier spirit that they gain from practicing tai chi.

Some exercises are difficult for people with diabetes: for example, if you have complications with your feet, it might be unsafe to take up jogging. If you are not well coordinated, you might find it too challenging to start playing golf or tennis. Also the competitiveness of many sports could increase your stress level. The Tai Chi for Diabetes program is designed to be easy and safe, and almost anyone with diabetes can learn it — but, since everyone's condition is different, check with your healthcare team before commencing this or any other tai chi program. You can practice it alone or with others.

Moderate exercise has been shown to improve the management of type 2 diabetes, and even prevent its onset. Being a gentle exercise, tai chi is a good option to consider. People who are stressed have poorer control of their diabetes, and because tai chi trains the mind to be more relaxed, it can improve the management of this condition.

If you go to a class to learn tai chi, you will be part of a social group. Many tai chi students enjoy the socialising and they find that the friendships they forge are invaluable. In one class there was a student who had poor diabetes control because she was not able to control her diet; that made her feel inadequate and she usually looked unhappy. One day she came to the tai chi class beaming. She said that her glucose control had improved. The student explained that at the previous week's class, one of her classmates reprimanded her for not sticking to the right diet. And for the next week, whenever she was going to break her diet, those words came back to her and she resisted. Tai chi does have more effect than being an exercise — the class creates a social bonding, almost like family. Students often say that you cannot choose your family but you can choose your tai chi family. This form of socialising is almost like group therapy. It is worth noting that many people who take up tai chi tend to be more serene and easy to be with. If you are not so serene, tai chi helps you get closer to being so.

At one level tai chi is a wonderful expression of the self and it helps to improve self-esteem and your sense of wellbeing. Feeling better about yourself helps you to cope with a chronic condition such as diabetes.

Complementary therapy

There is no doubt that Western medicine is most effective at treating diabetes, especially type 1: indeed, without insulin, people with type 1 diabetes could not survive. There is no proven alternative therapy that can replace insulin. Many complications of diabetes, especially acute conditions such as infections and hypoglycaemia, often require urgent Western medical care. But when it comes to type 2 diabetes and some of its complications that have no cure, such as arthritis and heart conditions, alternative therapy may provide help.

Many people with diabetes have considered using alternative therapies for their management. When used along with conventional treatments, these complementary therapies might improve your health and the quality of your life: the benefits of a number of alternative therapies are now well accepted by the medical establishment. It is most important that your healthcare team know about any therapy that you are using.

If the alternative therapy involves taking tablets, herbs or potions of any sort, be aware that natural material is not free of side effects — and *always* discuss this with your doctor. Remember, if any substance can do good to your body, it could also harm you. Many well-known pharmaceutical agents (drugs) are extracts from natural products — for example, digitalis, which makes the heart pump stronger and is a common ingredient in a medication for heart condition, comes from the foxglove. In a sense, there is no difference between so-called 'natural' herbs and prescribed drugs: whatever causes any effects on your body can also cause side effects.

Even non-invasive therapies, such as aromatherapy, relaxation therapy or exercise, may have side effects. For example, if you have a bad infection and you choose aromatherapy rather than conventional medicine, you could jeopardise your chance of recovery by not using antibiotics as soon as possible.

We recommend that you work with your healthcare team when you utilise any alternative therapy because any change in your body can affect your diabetes management. For example, if you are more relaxed, your blood glucose may be lowered: if you are receiving insulin or some medication and your glucose is too low, you can get more hypoglycaemia. Naturally, It is a good thing to have a lower glucose level as long as your healthcare team know about it and adjust the dosage of your medication accordingly.

If you are planning to use an alternative therapy, it is a good idea to try to find out if any scientific studies have been done on the therapy's efficacy (effectiveness) and safety.

Types of alternative therapies
Mind-body therapies
There are several kinds of mind-body practices that may relieve stress, pain, anxiety and depression and promote health. These use different approaches but are closely related in their results. They have been described as 'different doors that lead to the same room'.

- *Meditation* is a practice that develops calmness and insight. For example, concentration techniques help you calm your mind by focusing on the silent repetition of a word, a sound or the feel of your own breathing. This approach is taught in many stress-reduction programs. Reduction of stress can help diabetes control.
- *Biofeedback* uses electronic monitors to help you learn how to use your mind to affect and change specific body functions. It is effective for relaxation.
- *Visualisation* and *guided imagery* use the power of your imagination to take you to places or times when you are peaceful and healthy. These techniques are used to relieve pain, promote relaxation and change behaviour patterns. Athletes also use them to improve performance.
- *Hypnosis* is a concentration technique that focuses your mind on a specific action or thought. You can have someone lead you through this technique, or learn to do it yourself as *self-hypnosis*.
- *Relaxation exercises* help make you aware of tension and show you how to relieve it. They may include *breathing exercises* that use the connection between breath and emotions to teach relaxation and to energise.

- *Yoga* and *qigong* use gentle, precise movements coupled with breathing and concentration to exercise the body and calm and energise the mind.
- *Tai chi* uses movement in coordination with mental training, putting practitioners in a state almost like meditation. Studies have shown that it improves physical health, such as cardiovascular fitness, muscle strength, blood pressure and others. More importantly, tai chi helps the mind to be more balanced, serene and strong, as well as raises the spirit. Be aware that there are a number of forms of tai chi with significant differences between them. Be sure to consult your healthcare team about the right form of tai chi for you.

Herbs

Herbal therapy has been used by different cultures for thousands of years. Although, as yet, few herbs have been scientifically studied for their effect on diabetes, it is possible that there is a particular herb that could help lower blood pressure and even blood glucose. It is important to understand that some effects may not be desirable to your health. If you wish to use herb therapy, your healthcare team should know about it and monitor your condition more closely.

Dietary supplements

There are many false claims made about dietary supplements, some of which are useless or even dangerous. You should check with your dietitian, bringing a list of the exact components of the supplements you wish to try before using them.

Vitamins and *minerals* are essential for good health. A normal diet, including fresh fruit and vegetables, usually provides adequate supplies. However, this may not be possible for some people. A multivitamin supplement will ensure you are getting all the necessary nutrients. There is no evidence that mega-doses of particular vitamins or minerals help diabetes — and too much of some vitamins can be harmful. This too should be checked with your dietitian.

Acupuncture

Acupuncture originated in China thousands of years ago, and is based on the theory that qi (or life force) flows through the body along invisible channels, called meridians. When the flow of qi is blocked or out of balance, illness or pain results. Stimulation of specific points along the meridians can correct the flow of qi to restore or improve health. In acupuncture, hair-fine needles are inserted into the skin at precise points along the meridians. These can also be stimulated with heat and herbs (called moxibustion) and mild electrical current (electroacupuncture). Manual pressure (acupressure), magnets and special laser beams are sometimes used instead of needles.

Western scientists don't fully understand how acupuncture works — so far there is no evidence to support it helping blood-glucose control.

Homeopathy

Homeopathy is based on the idea that 'like cures like' and that very diluted amounts of a poison or other disease-causing substance can relieve the same symptoms that the larger dose causes. This concept resembles the de-sensitising therapy used to relieve allergy symptoms, or vaccination in which we are given a very mild case of the disease to put our immune system on guard. Millions of people worldwide believe in and use homeopathic remedies, but there is no solid scientific evidence that they do anything for diabetes. However, since the remedies are so very diluted, homeopathy is unlikely to cause any harm.

Beware of unsafe alternatives

When conventional medicine isn't doing well for your diabetes, it's tempting to turn to an alternative therapy. Most of these are unregulated and untested even for safety, so use your common sense and be careful. When your diabetes is not doing well, it does not mean you should try anything because your condition can get worse if you use unsafe alternatives.

- Always tell you doctor everything you are using or doing: some treatments could be harmful for you, or interfere with the prescription drugs you are taking. Many supplements, for example, are blood thinners and should be discontinued before you have surgery to avoid the risk of excessive bleeding.
- Be sure to buy from a reputable business that guarantees its products.
- Be especially careful about combining several herbs and supplements: you don't know what the overall effect might be.

And remember: just because it's natural doesn't mean its safe. Anything strong enough to help is strong enough to hurt. Nature also produces many of the most potent poisons.

PART II

CHAPTER 3

THE HEALING POWER OF TAI CHI

Originating in ancient China, tai chi is an effective exercise for health of mind and body. Although an art requiring great depth of knowledge and skill, it is easy to learn this specially designed program and you will soon experience its health benefits. Many will find that learning and enjoying tai chi continues throughout their lives

Almost anyone can learn the Tai Chi for Diabetes program. It's inexpensive and can be practiced anywhere. The movements are slow and gentle, and the degree of exertion can be easily adjusted, making it suitable for people of all levels of ability.

There are many styles and forms of tai chi, the major ones being Chen, Yang, Wu, Wu (they are different words in Chinese) and Sun. Each style has its own individual features, although most styles share similar essential principles.

These principles include: mind integrated with the body; control of the movements and breathing, and mental concentration. The central focus is to enable the qi or life force to flow smoothly and powerfully throughout the body. Total harmony of the inner and outer self comes from the integration of mind and body, achieved through the ongoing practice of tai chi.

What is tai chi?

Tai chi can be an exercise, an art or a tool. The ultimate aim of tai chi is to help us restore and improve the balance within ourselves and with the outside world. This unique and powerfully effective exercise system incorporates the ancient Chinese understanding of the universe, traditional Chinese medicine and traditional martial arts.

It is popular nowadays and you may have seen people in parks practicing this slow dance-like exercise — often with a focused intensity and serenity in their facial expressions. It is not difficult to be drawn to the beauty and naturalness of tai chi movements, especially when they are being executed among nature.

Its many health benefits and the enjoyment of practice are the reasons that tai chi has become more popular. Even people with chronic conditions who look at these gentle exercises think, 'yes, I can do that' — in contrast to the sweat and vigour of exercises in the gym. Tai chi has an intrinsic attraction and, after the initial learning period, people often become 'addicted' to it.

There are many unique features of tai chi: the slow and almost meditative movements, for example, and the circular or curve-like paths they follow. In nature, slowness complements fastness, and straight lines are balanced out with curves. Perhaps it is these features that bring us back to nature and help us to feel and understand our inner self — perhaps this is the main attraction of tai chi.

To a Westerner, tai chi is a very different form of exercise to most we are familiar with. Tai chi is derived from the observation of nature. In nature, there is balance of hardness and softness, light and darkness, movement and stillness. We need both physical and mental exercises to maintain health and balance: our bodies do well when they harmonise with nature.

The modern lifestyle has dramatically altered the balance of nature. The stress of modern life moves at such a fast pace, leaving no time to slow down and regenerate, and the means of transport has greatly decreased the amount of physical exercise we do. Tai chi allows our bodies to have that balance, allowing us time to get to know our inner selves. According to traditional Chinese medicine, when a human is in balance within him- or herself, she or he reaches health and longevity — and being in balance with nature means being healthier.

A great feature of tai chi is that it can be easily adapted and practiced by people with different abilities and with any physical disabilities — this is because, in tai chi, training focuses on the internal and its essential principle is to train people from the inside out.

'Inside' means the mind, the internal structure, the bones, the deep muscles and the internal organs. The internal training method uses your mind, which means that virtually anyone who is able to think can adapt tai chi as an exercise. The balance between internal and external is important: after all, you need to have a strong mind to help you to cope with life. The strong inside also means stronger internal organs, muscles and bones, giving you more stability and function. As many studies have shown, tai chi improves muscle strength, cardiovascular fitness and flexibility — all essential components for better health. We know that when the internal body becomes weak (and the mind, in cases such as depression), people will be more likely to get ill.

Tai chi helps to improve almost every aspect of health and it can be used as a tool for personal growth. If you have diabetes, it improves the health of your body and mind — and thus your condition. The specially designed program for diabetics offers a safe and easy way to use this tool.

If you wish to know more about the history of tai chi, see Dr Paul Lam and Nancy Kaye's *Tai Chi for Beginners and the 24 Forms* (see page 175).

What is Tai Chi for Diabetes?

There are many sets and forms of tai chi, with significant differences between them. Once you gain some knowledge of tai chi, you will find that, even among schools of similar origin, their forms can vary greatly: they can look significantly different in terms of variations of speed, physical exertion and means of expression.

Most tai chi forms are gentle, although some can be difficult for people with diabetes to learn — for example, the most popular Yang style with 108 moves may take an average learner, taking a lesson once a week, up to two years to learn. There are some forms that may have high risk for people with diabetes — for example the Chen style, which includes jumping in the air and stamping on the ground, could pose an extra risk.

People with diabetes will most likely prefer a tai chi set that carries

THE ADVANTAGES OF TAI CHI

These are some of many reasons so many people like tai chi.

- It can be done by just about anyone in any physical condition. You can begin or continue to do tai chi well into old age.

- It is inexpensive. Tai chi does not require any equipment, special clothing or environment. It can be done just about anywhere, outdoors or indoor, either alone or in a group. Classes generally are low cost. And once it is learned — from a book, video or class — it costs nothing to continue.

- The Tai Chi for Diabetes program is easy to learn. The movements can be adjusted to your ability and, with regular practice, you can gain better health and well being.

- It's easy to practice daily — you can do ten to twenty minutes a day or longer. It is easy to fit the program into your schedule.

- The more you progress, the more you enjoy it and the healthier you become. Tai chi is one activity where age doesn't matter: you don't regress as you grow older and you progress irrespective of age.

the minimum risk, delivers benefits quickly, is enjoyable and helps them to relax.

This special Tai Chi for Diabetes set is safe, easy to learn and is designed to be effective in preventing and controlling diabetes. It includes two tai chi styles: the Sun and Yang. The Sun style — characterised by a higher stance, agility and an emphasis on qigong (energy-cultivating exercises) — is powerfully effective for improving relaxation and focus. The Yang style, on the other hand, has some movements that involve more inner strength and greater exertion.

The program is designed with five levels of physical exertion: beginners start at the lowest level and gradually build up to the higher levels as their physical abilities improve. This is especially important for people with diabetes, because it minimises the risk of hypoglycaemia, as well as other complications. People with diabetes have six times more risk of having heart disease and often have poor balance because of arthritis and nerve damage to the feet. So the gradual increase in physical exertion lessens the chances of making these medical conditions worse.

Sun styles are more prominent in the first three levels, which are designed to help improve relaxation and generate more life energy. The fourth and fifth levels use more Yang-style movements and include the two key Yang movements: Waving Hands in the Cloud and Stroking Birds Tail. According to Yang Shau-zhong, one of the greatest Yang tai chi masters, these are the two most powerful forms in the style.

How does Tai Chi for Diabetes work?

The human body is designed to be active — an inactive lifestyle predisposes you to higher risk of many diseases. Most of us know that regular exercise is very important for good health. There is scientific evidence that people who exercise regularly are about 60 per cent less likely to develop type 2 diabetes — that is more than halving the risk. If you already have diabetes, regular exercise improves the control of your condition and reduces the risk of complications, leading to a better quality of life.

The word 'exercise' is often associated with sweating and puffing in a gymnasium. Many people with diabetes don't like exercise, especially with these sorts of mental images in the mind. And some exercises may not be appropriate for you — for example, jogging can be risky for those who have peripheral neuropathy (loss of nerve endings at the extremities, resulting in less feeling in the feet and hands) or some heart conditions.

Not only is it important to find an exercise that you can do safely, it is also very important to find one that you enjoy or can learn to enjoy. After all, in the long run, you usually stop doing things you don't enjoy. Tai chi offers a major advantage: it's intrinsically enjoyable; indeed, to many, it is a road to health and harmony. After the initial learning phase, of about three to six months, and becoming familiar with the rhythm and feel of tai chi, most people really enjoy it. And a great thing about tai chi is that it is not about competing — it is just for you. It makes you feel better about yourself. Practicing tai chi can be fun — and it makes you feel serene, healthier and happier.

If you live a sedentary life, chances are you don't like exercise because you don't enjoy doing it. It is very possible that you feel this way because you have not done well in the past with the exercises or sports you have tried, especially the competitive ones. It is a vicious circle — the less you exercise, the less coordinated you become, and the less proficient at learning and doing it, and hence the less you enjoy it.

The Tai Chi for Diabetes program is designed with this in mind. It will improve your coordination, you can progress at your own pace and there is no competitive grading. No matter what physical condition you are in, once you have learned Tai Chi for Diabetes and practice it regularly, your physical and mental health will improve. It's very likely that you will feel so good about yourself that you will want to continue tai chi for your lifetime.

Tai Chi for Diabetes and other exercises

An effective exercise should improve your muscle strength, cardio-vascular fitness and flexibility. It should also improve your mental health so that you are more relaxed and balanced. Tai Chi for Diabetes is designed to do these and more. It will help you to feel better about yourself and your condition. It is also designed to incorporate traditional Chinese medical theory to enhance its health benefits.

Tai chi is different from most Western exercises in the sense that the movements are slow. People who are used to the fast pace of modern life often find it difficult to slow down. They may say tai chi is too boring for them — but watching it is quite different from doing it. Once you get used to tai chi, the slowness represents peace and tranquility and it becomes a natural complement to, and a way to feel and appreciate, your body. Moving slowly allows you to connect your mind to your body and enhances focus. There are other patterns of movements, such as moving in a curve rather than a straight line, that are very different from Western practices. In fact, moving in a curve is a part of nature — almost all beautiful objects have a curve to them. Once you have got over the initial awkwardness, most will experience the intrinsic enjoyment of the feel and rhythm of tai chi. It usually takes three to six months to get used to the tai chi movements.

Many people really enjoy tai chi's slow, graceful movements and intrinsic tranquility. Although it can seem so effortless to people who never try it, it is in fact much more challenging than it appears. When you start learning tai chi, you might get frustrated that you cannot do the smooth and graceful movements quickly. It is good to be aware of this so that disappointment does not make you stop practicing. Tai chi is like a good wine: it gets better with maturity.

Tai Chi for Diabetes is designed to be easy to learn and quick to deliver health benefits. You don't have to do tai chi to a very high level before you gain health benefits: depending on how often you practice, many studies show students gaining benefits after only three months.

Some traditional teachers emphasise the martial arts aspect of tai chi and some use teaching methods that are not friendly to learners. If you want to learn with a teacher, it is important to look for one who understands your medical condition and is willing to work with your healthcare team.

All the available medical evidence on building muscular strength, flexibility and cardiovascular fitness has been incorporated into the Tai Chi for Diabetes program. It utilises slow, fluid movements combined with mental imagery and deep breathing to help you relax and strengthen your body. Scientific studies have shown tai chi to have beneficial effects on cardio-respiratory fitness, muscular strength, balance and peripheral circulation, and have shown tai chi to reduce tension and anxiety.

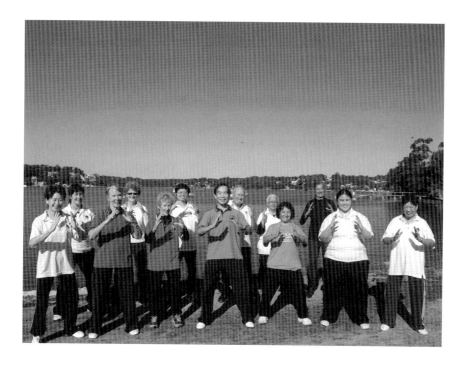

The power of the mind

Tai Chi for Diabetes enhances concentration, improves relaxation and uplifts the mood. Generally, the immense power of the mind has not been fully utilised. As one of the most effective mind-body exercises, tai chi teaches the student to harness the intrinsic energy from which he or she can attain greater self-control and empowerment.

Traditional Chinese medicine and qi

'Qi' is the life energy inside a person. Traditional Chinese medicine is based largely on the concept of qi, which is fundamental to most Eastern cultures. According to traditional Chinese medicine, diabetes is a deficiency of moisture and essence (yin) of the lung, spleen and kidney meridians. Enhancing qi in the appropriate meridians therefore improves diabetes. The Tai Chi for Diabetes program is designed to put emphasis on enhancing these meridians.

Designed to cultivate and enhance qi, tai chi encourages gentle and slow movements which stretch the body's meridians (energy channels along which qi travels) and keep them strong and supple. The rhythmic movements of the muscle, spine and joints pump energy through the whole body.

CHAPTER 4

GETTING READY

Before you start

- Be sure to check with your health professionals before you start, and if you develop any problem later. It is very important to read this chapter before continuing on to the next.
- Think about why you want to learn tai chi. Maybe it's for your health — physical, mental, or both. Whatever your reason, before you start on your journey of learning, define your goal. That way, you won't be just doing tai chi, you'll have something definite to work towards.
- Be prepared to practice regularly. Start with a time that is realistic for you — even just a few minutes — and build up to thirty to sixty minutes most days. Be sure to warm up before each practice session and do the cool-down exercises afterwards.
- As you practice, listen to your body. You should feel comfortable, not over-tired and never in pain.
- Wear loose, comfortable clothing and flat shoes. Dress in layers, so you can easily adjust when you get too hot or too cold.
- Be patient. As a tai chi novice, don't expect immediate satisfaction. It takes a while for tai chi to prove its powers.

Helping tai chi achieve your goal

If you've decided to give tai chi a try, you should realise that just *doing* tai chi won't do much for you. To reach your goal, you'll need to form a partnership with tai chi. The formula:

Motivation + tai chi = success

You may find the rhythm and feel of tai chi offers you a sense of peace and serenity that captures you straight away. Chances are you may also find tai chi is not as easy to learn as you expected. The seemingly effortless grace and gentle movements of tai chi do not come to learners over a few days.

It may be more challenging to move slowly than fast, especially if the movements are to be precise. Tai chi is different from most other exercises because its philosophy and essential principles are different from Western exercises. Faster is not always better — in fact, with the slow tai chi movements, it can take you to a tranquil place in your mind faster than fast-moving exercises. Once people get used to tai chi, the slowness become a natural place for peace and tranquility. Likewise, moving in a curve can be a faster way to get somewhere. Please keep these points in mind and give yourself time to settle in.

Most medical studies have shown the benefits of tai chi come to you within about three months. Long-term practice will give you even greater health benefits.

Regular practice is the major key to gaining significant benefits from tai chi. Here are some important practice tips:

- Set a regular practice time, so tai chi becomes part of your daily routine.
- When you start practice, work out a goal for the session — for example, to remember the sequence. Be sure to set a goal that is challenging but not over-challenging. Check the goal frequently as you practice. This will help you to be more focused and be in the flow.
- Make a schedule of when you expect to achieve how much — for example, if your goal is to lose weight, set a realistic target of, say, 2 kilograms per month.
- Try to practice with someone else, especially when you're feeling unmotivated.
- Be gentle with yourself. Stay within your comfort range for the level of exertion and length of your practice session.
- Do all movements slowly, continuously and smoothly. As you become more familiar with the movements, they will start to flow more easily and feel more graceful.
- Breathe slowly, naturally and easily. As you become used to doing

the moves, try to coordinate them with your breathing, as instructed. Return to your natural breathing if you find this is too forced.

- Gradually build up the length and number of practice sessions, aiming for about thirty to sixty minutes for most days. A simple indication of how long your first practice sessions should be is the length of time you can walk comfortably at a steady pace.

And a few important practice precautions:

- Continue your session only for as long as you feel comfortable. Listen to your body and rest when you start to feel tired, in pain, or lose concentration.
- Check with your doctor or healthcare team before you start the program. Bring this book to show them. Explain that at the beginning the physical exertion level is similar to slow walking and that very gradually it will progress to the level of a brisk walk. Ask and write down any precautions your healthcare team asks you take.
- If your knees become tired, stiff or painful in the bent position, stand up between movements. As your muscles become stronger, you will be able to stay comfortably in the squatting position for longer.
- Avoid practicing in a place that is too hot, too cold or is windy.
- After practicing, avoid subjecting yourself to an extreme change of temperature — for example, don't immediately go from a very hot practice environment to an air-conditioned area. And when you're hot from practicing, don't drink cold or chilled drinks: subjecting the body to sudden and extreme change could cause harm — a fact that is well known in Chinese traditional medicine and is now also recognised by Western medicine.
- Practice in an area that is clear of obstacles and has a non-slippery surface with no loose mats or rugs.
- Don't practice when you're very hungry, immediately after a big meal or when you're very upset.

- Don't continue doing any movement that is painful or causes you discomfort. If you experience chest pains, shortness of breath or dizziness, or if additional pain in your joints persists, stop and consult your health professionals.

Dress for the part

What should you wear to practice tai chi? The key word here is *comfort*. Wear loose, comfortable clothes and flat shoes. For everyday practice, clothing made of cotton is ideal because it allows your skin to breathe and it absorbs sweat. Although stretchy clothing such as leotards allow for free movement, it isn't good for tai chi because it sticks closely to the skin, inhibiting the flow of qi. (Qi travels along its meridians, which are close to the surface of the skin.) Also, avoid elastic around your waist and pant leg, because, again, this might restrict the flow of qi, as well as the blood flow.

It is a good idea to dress in layers. You might be cold when you start practicing, especially in winter, but if you work up a sweat, you can remove some layers. Layers are necessary in summer, too, in case you get too hot but also if a sudden wind comes up or if it gets colder.

Barefoot or with shoes?

Shoes can give you good support, help your balance and protect your feet if the ground is uneven or dirty. Also, if your feet get cold, the flow of qi could be impeded. If you have diabetes, your feet are more likely to have infection or loss of sensation, so you should protect your feet with good shoes.

The ideal practice shoes should:

- feel comfortable and soft
- be lightweight
- have broad base support in the sole to help you balance

- have shock-absorbent pads in the sole to minimise injury
- not be too tight
- have good ventilation.

Lace-up shoes such as the martial arts shoes made by Adida or New Balance are suitable, as long as they are comfortable for your feet. The traditional Chinese-made flat-bottom cotton cloth shoes are also suitable. In recent years, China has come out with different types of martial arts shoe that have a broadened base. They vary widely in quality, so take care to choose ones that fulfil the above criteria.

Ready, set, go …

You've set your goal. You've read the practice instructions (see page 58 on). You're even outfitted for your adventure in the art of tai chi. But before you turn the pages to begin your warm-ups, there's one more thing we suggest you need: patience — with tai chi and with yourself.

When you first begin, tai chi might seem easy, but the more you practice, the more you'll be aware of the challenges tai chi presents. That's where patience comes in. Don't expect immediate satisfaction. Don't be disappointed if you don't feel the picture of health after only a few days. And, above all, don't expect perfection. Nobody does tai chi perfectly — and therein lies the ongoing challenge of the art.

Some beginners might feel strange or even awkward when doing tai chi, particularly people who are used to fast-moving sports and moving in a straight line. In contrast, tai chi is slow, its movements curved and soft. Also the concept of internal might seem foreign. But rest assured that once you get used to all these differences, you won't feel awkward. Instead, you'll be hooked on the gentle movements that contain immense power. We suggest you give yourself at least three months, preferably six, to get used to these new concepts.

TAI CHI AND MEDICAL CONDITIONS

If you have any medical conditions, be sure to check with your healthcare team and let your tai chi instructors know. Below are some precautions you should take (in conjunction with your healthcare team's advice).

Hypoglycaemia

One of the significant dangers for people with diabetes who undertake exercise is hypoglycaemia (see chapter 1).

Exercise consumes a high level of energy and therefore blood glucose can be depleted rapidly. The body has an efficient system to regulate blood glucose so that it stays in the right range. However, as medication or injectable insulin aims to lower blood glucose, it may interfere with the body's regulatory system and cause hypoglycaemia. This is why you should let your doctor know what kind of exercise you're doing, and follow the doctor's advice and precautions.

Knee bends for people with arthritis

Many people suffer from arthritis in the knee joints. Tai chi requires bent knees and maintaining the same height throughout the set of forms. This can cause too much stress on the joints, especially for beginners. While one of the goals of tai chi is to keep the knees bent at the same height, you should work up to that very slowly (over months or even years). Stand up between movements to avoid excess stress to the knees.

Hip replacement

If you have had a hip replacement, you should avoid moving your foot across the midline. During the replacement surgery, your nerves responsible for the opposite side of the body could have been cut, thus affecting your ability to feel the position of your body. This, in turn, could affect your balance if your foot crosses the midline.

Steps 1 to 3

Warming up and cooling down

To help you remember the steps, we've designed Step 1 with *one* exercise, Step 2 with *two* stretches for six parts of the body, Step 3 with *three* exercises. Start by learning Steps 1 to 3, taking your time and practicing until you're comfortable with these three steps. They're gentle, easy-to-remember warming-up, stretching and cooling-down exercises. When you're ready to advance beyond Step 3, keep in mind that you should always start with Steps 1 and 2 to warm up and prepare your body. You should finish with Step 3, the cooling-down exercises, to loosen up and avoid injury.

Focus on the feel and rhythm of tai chi and don't worry too much about minor details.

If you happen to have a physical disability that prevents you from doing the exercises and movements to the full range, follow the instructions only to the extent that you remain within your comfort zone and visualise yourself doing the movements to their full range. Let's say, for example, that you've suffered a stroke and can't move your left leg. Visualise that your left leg is moving to its full extent as you're sitting and moving other parts of the body. Studies have shown that people can improve their abilities with visualisation.

Step 1: warm up — one exercise to start the blood circulating.

Step 2: stretching — two exercises for six parts of the body to prepare your body for tai chi.

Step 3: cooling down — three exercises to do at the conclusion to enhance your flexibility and prevent injury.

Lesson plan

We have provided you with a lesson plan based on a thirty-minute lesson. If you have only ten minutes or are unable to exercise for half an hour because of your physical condition, do only part of the lesson. The plan is a guide only. Do use your discretion and adjust it according to your own physical ability and learning speed. Remember, it's better to be slow and learn well, rather than attempting to learn the entire program quickly and missing out the important principles. Also the length of time to exercise is not set in stone. Keep in mind, five minutes of exercise are better than none.

After a session spent learning material — a 'learning lesson' — plan to spend approximately five practice sessions to become familiar and comfortable with the moves, and only then move on to the next lesson — for example, have one learning lesson on Monday and a practice session every day for one week, then start the next learning lesson next week. Try to practice daily, or at least most days.

Familiarising yourself with the first three steps might take one to three learning lessons.

Once you have familiarised yourself with the first three steps you can start learning Qigong for Diabetes. Use one to two lessons to learn part 1, Stationery Qigong, and the same time for part 2, Moving Qigong.

The next stage is the basic eleven-movement set, which is the core of the Tai Chi for Diabetes program. A rough guide is to use one learning lesson per movement, although difficult movements, such as Waving Hand in the Cloud, may take two or three.

You can continue to practice the Qigong for Diabetes and the eleven-movement set for as long as you wish in order to gain better health, improve your condition and to reach a higher level of tai chi. However if you have practiced for at least three months and wish to move to something more challenging, then consider starting the advanced nine-movement set.

Level of physical exertion

This program is designed with five levels of physical exertion to minimise any potential complications. Start with Level 1 and practice for a length of time until you become physically comfortable and fit before moving on to the next level. Consult your healthcare team if you have any doubt.

- *Level 1:* Steps 1 to 3 warm-up and cooling-down exercises: You can start doing these sitting down if you don't feel comfortable doing them standing up. If you are practicing these while sitting, be sure to visualise the rest of your body moving as completely as shown.

- *Level 2:* Stationary Qigong for diabetes.

- *Level 3:* Moving Qigong for diabetes.

- *Level 4:* Basic eleven-movement set.

- *Level 5:* Advanced nine-movement set.

STEP 1: WARM-UP EXERCISES

For about two minutes, walk around, gently shaking your hands and legs, and clenching and unclenching your hands. This loosens your body and joints and starts the blood circulating in preparation for the exercises that follow.

STEP 2: STRETCHING EXERCISES

Tai chi principles are integrated into these exercises. Practicing them regularly will enhance your flexibility and tune up your muscles.

- Do all movements slowly, continuously and smoothly.
- Move well within your comfort range. The first time you do a movement, stretch to only 70 per cent of your normal range — increase that range gradually.
- When appropriate, do both sides.
- Do each stretch three to five times. It doesn't matter which side you do first.
- If you have any difficulty balancing, use a chair or the wall for support.
- We're going to gently stretch six parts of the body — neck, shoulders, spine, hips, knees and ankles— with two stretches for each body part. It might help you to remember them by knowing we are working from the top down, starting with the neck and ending at the ankles. It is quite all right if you prefer to work from the bottom up.
- Unless otherwise specified, keep your feet a shoulder-width apart.

NECK

1. HEAD DOWN

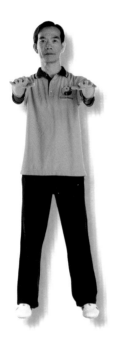 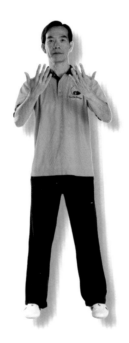 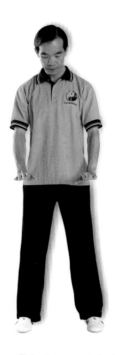

As you inhale, bring both hands up slowly, imagining your wrists are being lifted by two balloons.

Turn your palms so that your fingers are pointing upward. Bring them toward your chest and move your chin (or your head) backward gently.

Exhaling, push both hands outward, extending them in front of you, and then press your hands down slowly and gently. At the same time, slowly bring your head down toward your chest.

2. TURNING HEAD

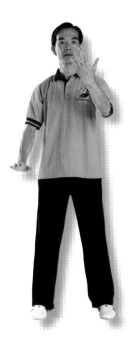 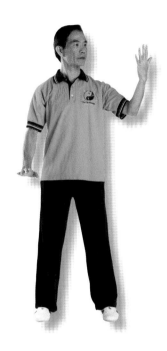

Lift up both hands as in the previous exercise, then turn your left hand so that its fingers are pointing up and the palm is facing you. At the same time, gently push the right hand down so that it is near the hip with the palm facing down. Look at your left palm.

Move your left hand to the left, turning your head slowly to the left and keeping your eyes on your palm. Then come back to face the front. Change palms so that your right palm is now facing you and the left is down near the left hip. Turn to the right while looking at the right palm.

SHOULDERS

1. SHOULDER ROLL

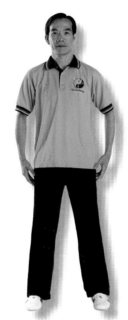

Roll shoulders gently forward three times and then backwards three times.

2. GATHERING QI

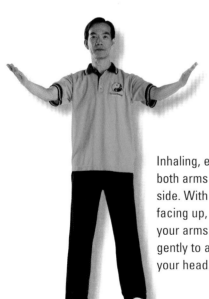

Inhaling, extend both arms to the side. With palms facing up, move your arms up gently to above your head.

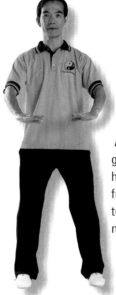

As you exhale, gently press your hands down in front of your body to below your navel.

SPINE

HEAVEN AND EARTH

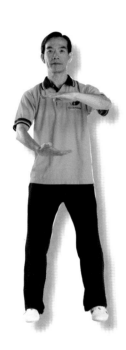

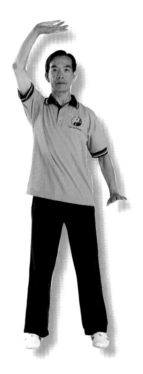

Hold your hands in front, one above the other, as though you're carrying a large beach ball. Inhale.

Exhaling, push the top hand up as though your palm is pushing against the ceiling. At the same time, push the other hand down by your side, and imagine stretching your spine gently. Repeat the exercise with other hand.

SPINE TURN

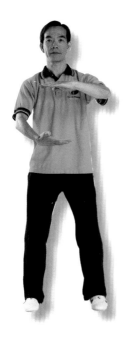 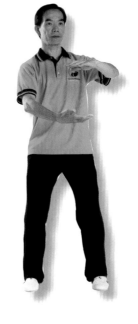

Hold your hands in front, one above the other, as though you're carrying a large beach ball. Left hand on top.

Bend knees slightly, turn your waist gently to the left. Then change hands, putting the right hand on top and turn to the right. Keep your back upright and supple and be sure to turn no more than 45 degrees from the front (draw an imaginary line vertical to the knee and don't let your hands move pass this line).

HIP

1. FORWARD STRETCH

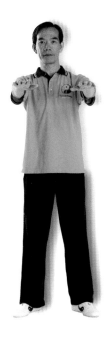

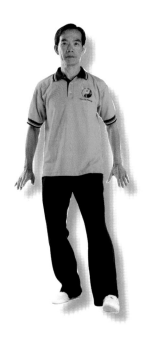

Start with hands in front, knees slightly bent.

Place your left heel out in front of you and push both hands back to help balance.

2. SIDE STRETCH

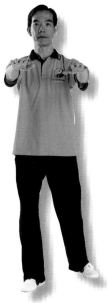

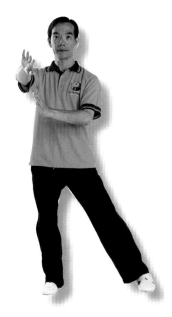

Step backwards so that your left foot is resting on its toes, while stretching your hands forward to about shoulder height for better balance. Repeat with the right foot.

An easy alternative: Place your left foot on the ground parallel to the right foot before stepping backwards.

Bending your knees slightly, push your hands to the left side as though you're pushing against a wall. At the same time, stretch the right foot out sideways. Maintain upright posture and stretch only as far as comfortable. Repeat the exercise on the other side.

KNEES

1. KICK

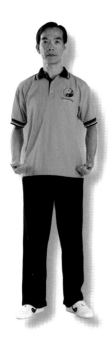

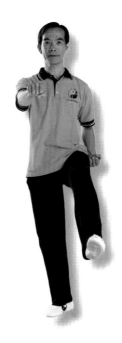

Make loose fists, palm side up, resting at the sides of the hips. Bend your knees slightly.

Alternative: Stretch out one foot so that the toes touch the ground, and then bring it back.

Stretch out one foot (like a kicking motion, but slowly and gently). At the same time, punch out gently with the opposite fist, turning it palm down. Bring your arm and leg back in. Repeat on the other side.

2. STEP FORWARD

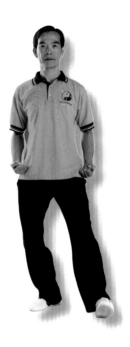

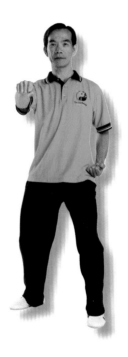

Hold your fists next to your hips as in the previous exercise, bend your knees slightly and step forward with one foot.

Shift your weight on to the front leg and. as your body moves forward, punch out with the opposite fist. Bring your arm and leg back. Repeat on the other side.

ANKLES

1. TAPPING

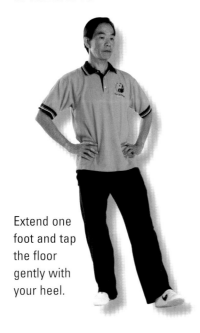

Extend one foot and tap the floor gently with your heel.

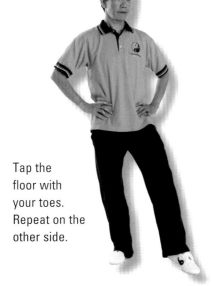

Tap the floor with your toes. Repeat on the other side.

2. ROTATION

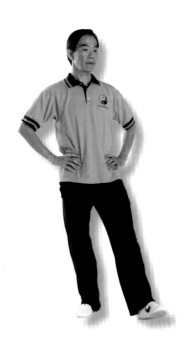

Lift up the heel of one foot, point the toes down and gently rotate your foot in one direction three times, and then in the other direction three times. Repeat exercise using the other foot.

Alternative: Turn your foot inwards and outwards several times, avoiding over-stretching by not putting any weight on the turning foot. Repeat exercise using the other foot.

STEP 3: COOLING-DOWN EXERCISES

These exercises are to be used after you complete your tai chi session. You should learn them now so that you can do them after your very first lesson. These exercises will help to enhance your flexibility, relax your muscles and prevent injury.

1. PUNCHING THIGH

2. TENSE AND RELAX

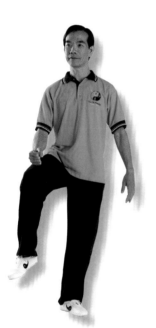

Inhaling, clench your hands, gently contract the muscles of your body, and stand on your toes if you can.

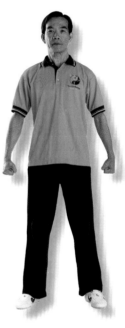

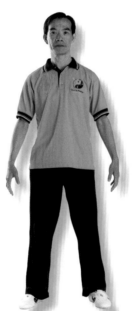

Lift your thigh to a comfortable height and gently punch it. Repeat with the other leg.

Exhale, letting everything relax.

3. GATHERING QI

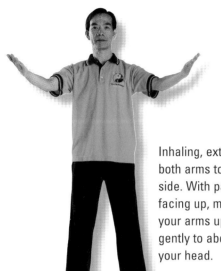

Inhaling, extend both arms to the side. With palms facing up, move your arms up gently to above your head.

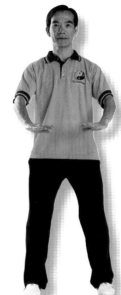

As you exhale, gently press your hands down in front of your body to below your navel.

Note: These are the same as for the second stretching exercise for the shoulder (see page 82).

PART III

CHAPTER 5

THE TAI CHI FOR DIABETES PROGRAM

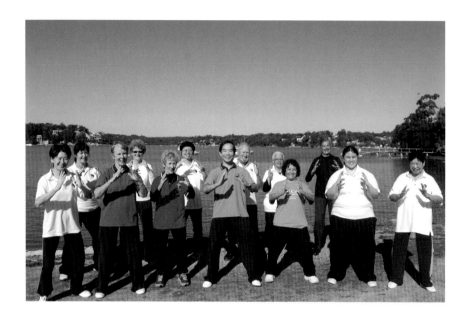

Qigong for diabetes

Qigong is an ancient Chinese practice that enhances health and relaxation. Yes, tai chi does that too. There are numerous types of qigong, whereas tai chi is an exercise that incorporates qigong as its core strength. A good way to look at this is that tai chi is an advanced and unique form of qigong.

Qi is the life energy within a person — indeed, according to Chinese medicine, qi is life. It flows through specific channels, called energy channels or meridians — the same meridians an acupuncturist uses (acupuncture is based on the same concept of qi) — and performs many functions, such as moving the blood, lymphatic fluid and energy around the body.

A person with strong qi will be healthy and live a long life. Each of us is endowed at birth with essential qi. That essential qi combines with the qi absorbed in the digestive system from food and water and the qi extracted from the air you breathe to form the vital life energy of the body. The storage house of qi is the dan tian, an area situated three finger-breadths below the belly button.

The concept of qi is fundamental to Chinese medicine. Practitioners believe that personal qi is related to the qi of the environment and the universe. Qi becomes stronger when you are in harmony with your environment, practice good nutrition, exercise regularly, and enjoy mental tranquility.

'Gong' means 'a method of exercise that requires a great deal of time to do well.' Although numerous forms of qigong exist, it is basically the practice of cultivating qi. It consists of special breathing exercises and meditation, sometimes integrated with movement. Tai chi incorporates qigong as an integral part of its practice — indeed, the internal power of tai chi is the qi.

When you practice qigong exercises, most of which have simple movements, you can focus on your inner self without having to think too much about the different movements. This concentration on mental imaging and relaxation will improve your tai chi and will help you to incorporate qi into the movements.

Tai chi, which is often called 'meditation in motion', contains many elements of qigong and is one of the most effective exercises for cultivating qi.

The Sun style, which constitutes half of this program, contains deep and powerful qigong. The gentle and slow movements open up your energy channels and keep them strong and supple; the rhythmic movements of the muscle, spine and joints pump energy through the whole body, and the deep concentration calms and unites the body, mind and spirit.

The Qigong for Diabetes program

Created especially for this program, this is based on traditional qigong and Sun-style tai chi. The exercises help you to relax and to prepare your mind and body for the tai chi set. They are effective at cultivating qi and enhancing your tai chi with regular practice.

1. STATIONARY QIGONG

OPEN AND CLOSE

Stand with your body upright but relaxed, with your feet slightly apart and knees relaxed. Look straight ahead, tuck in your chin slightly and relax your shoulders. At the same time, stand tall without being tense.

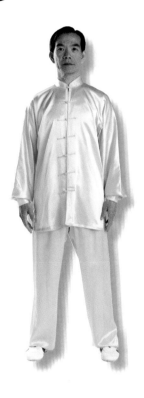

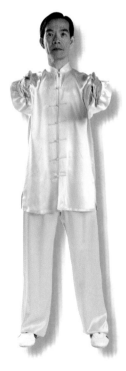

Breathing in, slowly bring both hands up to shoulder height, with the palms facing each other. At the centre of the palm there is an acupuncture point Lao Gong, which is the energy centre in the upper limb: when the two acupuncture points in both palms are facing each other, the flow of qi is enhanced.

Bend your knees slowly and slightly — if you look down and cannot see your toes, then you are bending too deeply. Bring both hands to the front of your chest: this is called the Praying Position (there is no religious meaning behind this name — it is just a way to describe the appearance of the position).

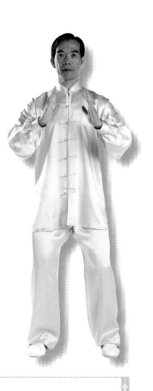

MAGNETIC FORCE

For Open and Close, as you open your hands, imagine there is a gentle magnetic force between the palms, preventing you from moving them so you have to gently pull them apart. As you push your hands towards each other, imagine the magnetic force working in reverse so that you have to gently push them closer.

Open: breathing in, slowly open your hands to shoulder width. As you inhale, visualise air entering your nose slowly, travelling past your windpipe and gently filling your lungs and then your abdomen. If your knee feels tired, straighten slowly at the same time.

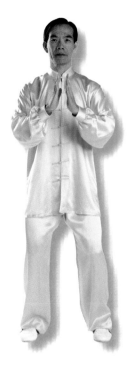

Close: breathing out slowly, push your hands towards each other. As you exhale, visualise air being expelled slowly from your abdomen and lungs, through your windpipe and nose. Bend your knees slightly if you have straightened them in the previous movement.

After doing the Open and Close exercises three times, bring your right hand down closer to the chest with the palm turned upward. At the same time, push your left palm forward from your shoulder and turn it down.

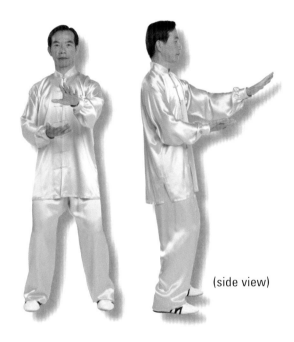

(side view)

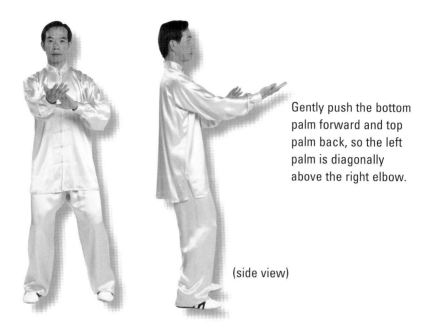

Gently push the bottom palm forward and top palm back, so the left palm is diagonally above the right elbow.

(side view)

Roll both arms up and over, as though both your hands are holding a large rolling pin; roll the arms upside down so that their positions are reversed with the top hand now at the bottom and bottom hand on top.

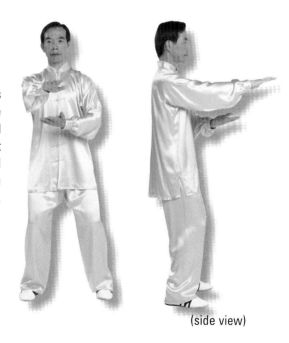

(side view)

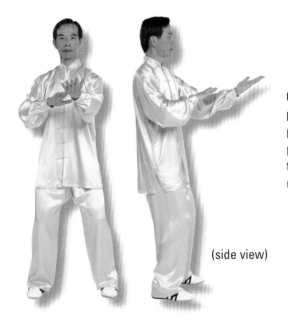

Gently push the bottom palm forward and the top palm back, so that the right palm is diagonally facing the left elbow. Repeat these movements three times.

(side view)

Bring both hands in front of the chest. Do Open and Close once.

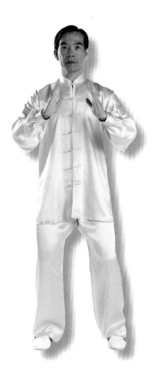

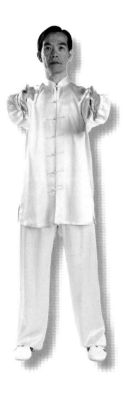

Slowly stretch
hands forward.

Lower your hands slowly
and stand up slowly
at the same time.

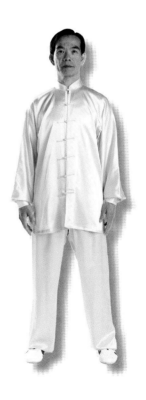

2. MOVING QIGONG

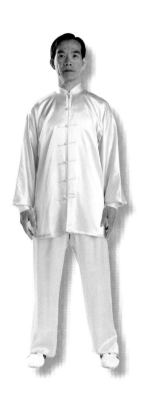

Preparation 1

Start from the
beginning position of
the Stationary Qigong.

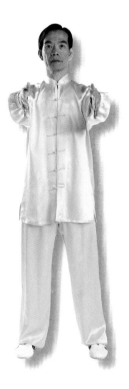

Preparation 2

Bring hands up.

Preparation 3

Do Open and Close three times.

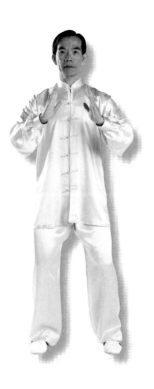

Bring the right hand back with palm facing up, and gently push left hand forward. At the same time, step forward with your left foot. Your left toes are pointing, at about a 60-degree angle, outwards.

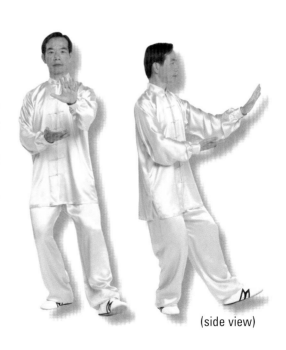

(side view)

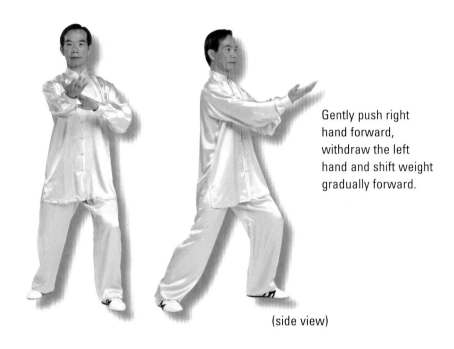

Gently push right hand forward, withdraw the left hand and shift weight gradually forward.

(side view)

Turn both palms upside down and step forward with your right foot.

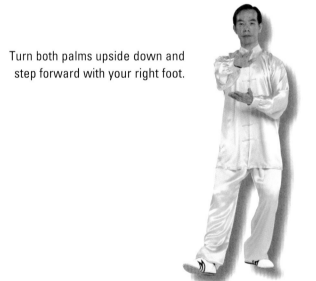

Shift weight forward and push left palm forward.

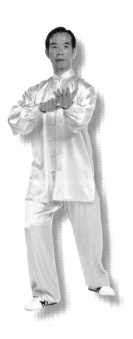

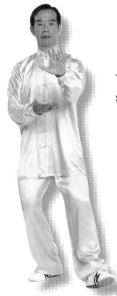

Turn both palms upside down and step forward with your left foot.

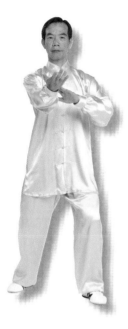

Continue to do the five movements of Moving Qigong several times. Then bring both hand to front of chest, feet parallel.

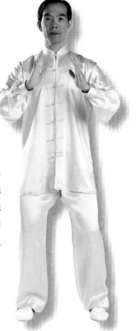

Do Open and Close once. Then push hands forward and bring hands down on the side and slowly stand up.

The dan tian breathing method

You can practice the breathing method either sitting or standing upright, or even lying down. Be aware of holding the correct upright and supple posture. Put your left hand on your abdomen just above the belly button and your right hand beside your hip with your index and middle fingers just above the groin. Concentrate on your lower abdomen and the pelvic floor muscle.

When you inhale, expand your lower abdominal area — allow it to bulge out a little. As you exhale, gently contract the pelvic floor muscles under the lower abdomen. Feel the contraction of the muscle under the index and middle fingers of your right hand, keeping the area above your belly button as still as possible (use your left hand to feel if there is any movement — it is nearly impossible not to move at all). Contract the pelvic floor muscles gently, so gently that it's almost like you're just thinking about it. Or imagine you are bringing your pelvic floor half a centimetre closer to your belly button. A stronger contraction would move the area above your belly button, which is less effective.

DAN TIAN BREATHING

This breathing method is a modification of traditional qigong, based on modern medical research into the deep stabiliser muscles (internal muscles that support the spine). Based on tai chi principles, sinking your qi to the dan tian enhances qi power, which in turn improves internal 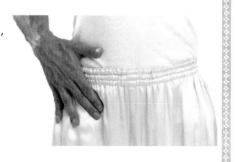 energy. The scientifically proven method of strengthening the deep stabilisers is incorporated into the breathing method, making this easier and more effective at enhancing qi. It can be incorporated into all your qigong and tai chi movements.

The basic set

This is the core of the program. Practice it regularly with the Qigong for Diabetes. It is well balanced and complete by itself, and you can continue to progress with tai chi and your health by practicing this and Qigong for Diabetes

If you wish to work on more challenging forms, you can start the advanced set (see page 136 on). It is recommended that you practice the Qigong and basic set for at least three months before moving on.

The flow chart opposite will help you remember the direction and movements of the set. You can purchase a wall chart with all the movements to help you during practice (see Resources, pages 174).

1. Commencement Movement.
2. Open and Close Hands.
3. Waving Hands in the Cloud (left, x 3)
4. Open and Close Hands.
5. Fair Lady Working at the Shuttle.
6. Open and Close Hands.
7. Toes Kicks (left and right).
8. Open and Close Hands.
9. Waving Hands in the Cloud (right, x 3)
10. Open and Close Hands.
11. Closing Movement.

STARTING POSITION

Stand with your body upright but relaxed — feet together, knees loose, eyes looking forward, chin tucked in, shoulders relaxed. Cleanse your mind.

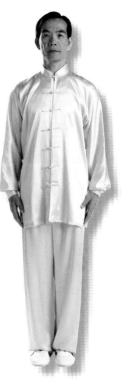

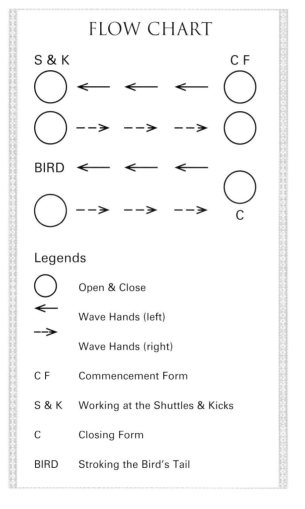

FLOW CHART

S & K   C F

○ ← ← ← ○

○ --→ --→ --→ ○

BIRD ← ← ←

○ --→ --→ --→ ○
                                          C

Legends

○   Open & Close

←   Wave Hands (left)

--→   Wave Hands (right)

C F   Commencement Form

S & K   Working at the Shuttles & Kicks

C   Closing Form

BIRD   Stroking the Bird's Tail

MOVEMENT 1

COMMENCEMENT MOVEMENT

Lift your left foot just above the ground, heel first, then place it on the ground approximately a shoulder-width apart from and parallel to the right foot. As you step down, place your toes down first. Visualise yourself as a string with both ends of the string gently stretched out, or simply standing upright without being tense.

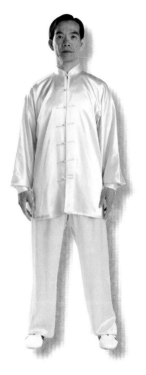

MOVEMENT 2

OPEN AND CLOSE HANDS

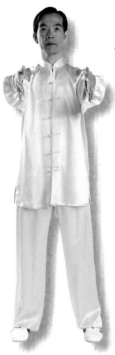

1. Breathing in, slowly bring both hands up to shoulder height, with palms facing each other.

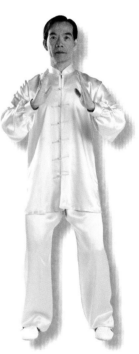

2. Slowly bend your knees slightly. Bring both hands to the front of the chest to the Praying Position.

3. Breathing in slowly, open your hands slowly to the width of your shoulders. As you open your hands, imagine there is a gentle magnetic force between the palms so that you have to gently pull them apart. Visualise air entering your nose slowly, travelling past your windpipe and gently filling your lungs and then the abdomen.

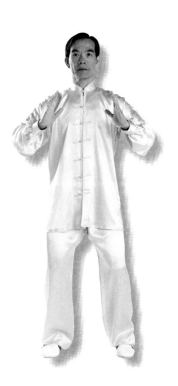

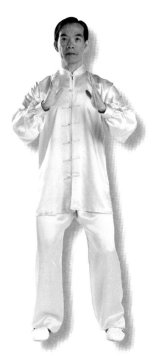

4. Breathing out slowly, push hands towards each other to head width. Imagine the magnetic force between your hands working reverse so that you have to gently push them closer. Visualise air being expelled slowly from your abdomen and lungs, through your windpipe and nose.

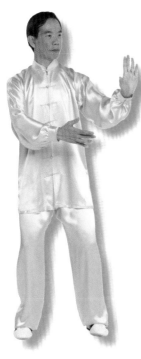

MOVEMENT 3

WAVING HANDS IN THE CLOUD (LEFT)

Stationary Movements

You will learn the upper body movements, then the steps for the lower body; you can combine them together in one movement. Once you have learned the complete movement, you don't need to split up the upper and lower body in your practice.

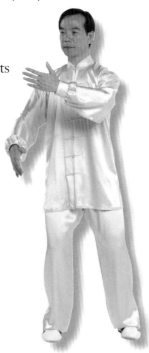

Upper body movements

1. Turn your torso slightly to the right, and bring your left hand up and right hand down below the left — almost as though you are embracing someone on the right side of your body.

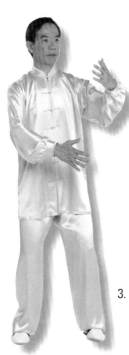

2. Turn your waist gently and bring both hands to the left.

3. Slowly turn the left palm out, taking care to keep your fingers angled upwards as you turn.

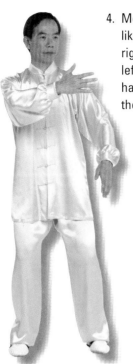

4. Moving in a gentle curve-like motion, bring your right hand up and your left hand down. As the left hand moves down, turn the palm to face inward.

5. Turn your waist gently and bring both hands to the right.

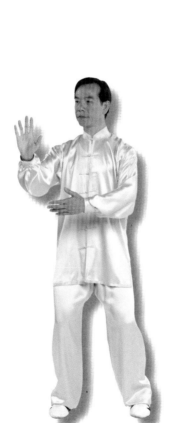

6. Slowly turn the right palm out, take care to keep your fingers pointing diagonally upwards as you turn.

Repeat steps 1 to 6 three times

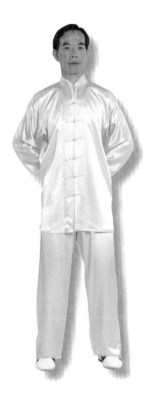

The steps

1. Start with your feet parallel and separated by your shoulder width, hands behind your back or on your hips and knees slightly bent.

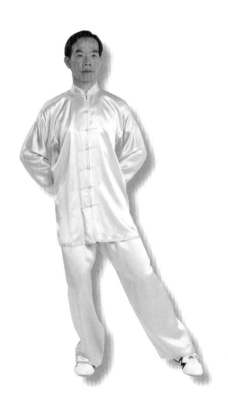

2. Transfer your weight on to your right foot. Lift up the left heel and then the entire left foot just above the ground. Step out with left foot to a distance comfortable to you —about half a step is a good distance. Start with a short length, and as you become stronger with regular practice, you can slowly increase the distance.

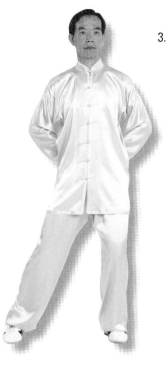

3. Transfer weight
   to the left foot.

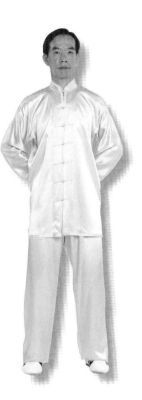

4. Step right foot in
   closer to the left. The
   distance between
   both feet should be at
   least two fists wide
   — if your feet are
   any closer, you might
   become unstable.

Repeat steps 1 to 4 three times from the Praying Position.

PRECAUTIONARY NOTE

If you are comfortable, keep both your knees slightly bent at the
same degree while doing this movement. However, if you feel
any strain, stand up in between each step; as your knees become
stronger with practice, you can slowly increase the degree of knee
bend (although you should never bend them so much that you
cannot see your toes when you look down — this means that if you
draw a vertical line between your knee cap and the tip of your toes,
the knee should never go over this line).

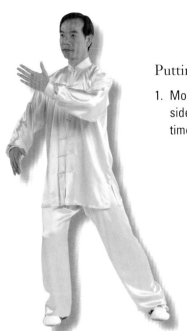

Putting it all together

1. Move both hands to the right side of your body. At the same time, step out with left foot.

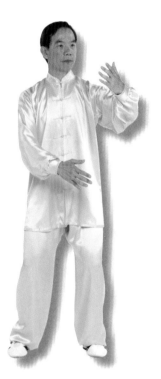

2. Move hands to the left and step in with the right foot.

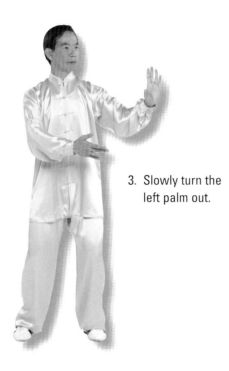

3. Slowly turn the
   left palm out.

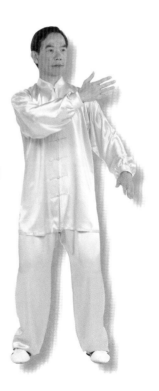

4. Bring your left hand
   down and right
   hand up slowly.

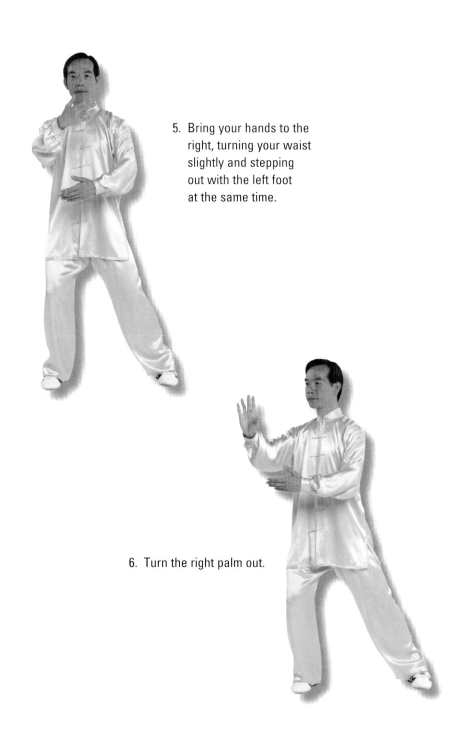

5. Bring your hands to the right, turning your waist slightly and stepping out with the left foot at the same time.

6. Turn the right palm out.

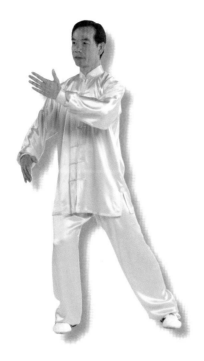

7. Bring your right hand down and left hand up slowly.

Repeat steps 1 to 6 three times.

MOVEMENT 4

OPEN AND CLOSE HANDS

Bring both hands gently to the front to the Prayer Position, and repeat Movement 2.

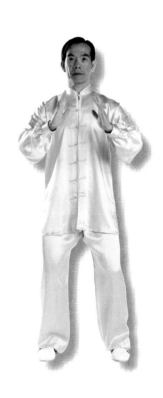

MOVEMENT 5

FAIR LADY WORKING AT THE SHUTTLE

1. Transfer weight to the right foot. Lift up your left hand and bring your right hand closer to the chest, with both palms facing out. Bring left foot closer to the right.

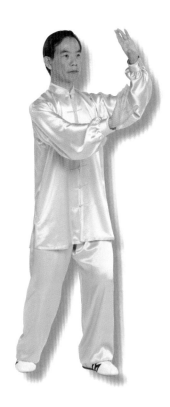

2. Step forward with your left foot at an angle of 45 degrees (10.30 on a clock if you start facing 12 o'clock). At the same time, move your left hand further up and your right hand slightly closer to the body.

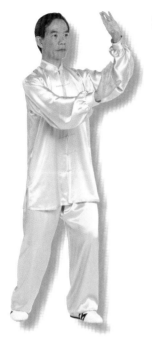

3. With both palms out, slowly move your left hand across and over the left side of your head as though you are protecting your head, and push your right hand gently forward. At the same time, shift your weight forward and bring your right foot closer to the left, landing with the ball of your foot on the ground and heel just above ground.

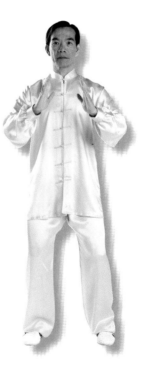

4. Step back with your right foot, then the left. At the same time, bring both hands back to form the Praying Position.

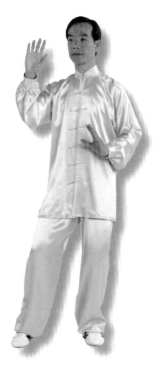

5. Transfer your weight to the left foot. At the same time, lift up your right hand and bring the left hand closer to the chest with both palms facing out. Bring your right foot closer to the left.

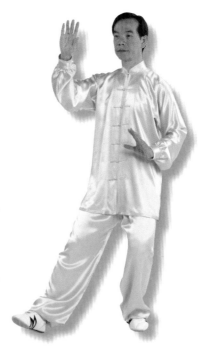

6. Take a step forward with your right foot to an angle of 45 degrees (1.30 position on a clock, if you start facing 12 o'clock). At the same time, move your right hand further up and your left hand slightly closer to your body.

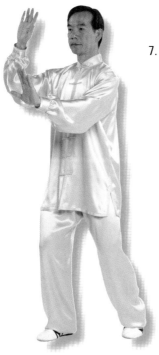

7. Move your right hand over your head as though you are protecting your head, and push your left hand forward. At the same time, shift your weight forward and bring your left foot closer to the right.

MOVEMENT 6

OPEN AND CLOSE HANDS

Slowly bring both hands in front of your chest to form the Prayer Position and repeat Movement 2.

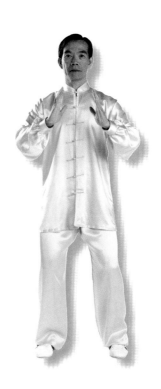

MOVEMENT 7

TOE KICKS (LEFT AND RIGHT)

The hand movements and the kicking movements are learned separately, then the upper and lower body movements are combined. Once you have learned the complete movement, you don't need to split up the upper and lower body in your practice.

Hand movements

1. From the Prayer Position, turn both palms slowly to face out.

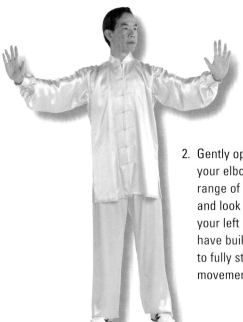

2. Gently open your hands outward by extending your elbow joint to 70 per cent of its full range of movement with fingers pointing up, and look at the tip of the middle finger of your left hand. All tai chi movements should have build-in reserves — it is not desirable to fully stretch any joints; at the end of this movement, the elbow is still slightly bent.

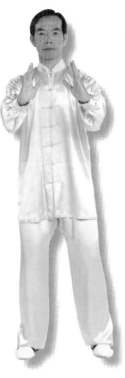

3. Bring hands back to the Praying Position.

4. Gently open your hands outwards about 70 per cent, with fingers pointing up, and look at the tip of the middle finger of your right hand.

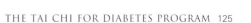

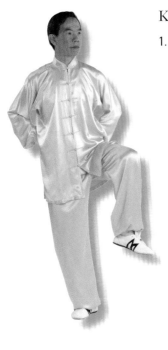

Kicking movements

1. Place your hands on your back or your hips, transfer your weight on to the right foot and gently lift up your left knee.

2. Kick out with the left leg slowly. Be sure to only kick to a height that is comfortable for you.

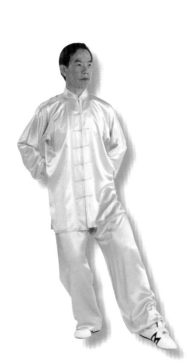

Alternative: If you have any difficulty balancing with one foot, simply lift your knee up a little, step your left foot forward and touch down on the heel.

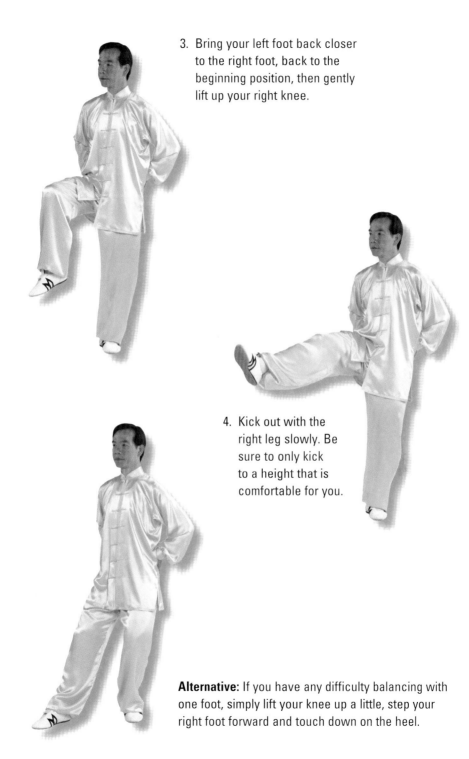

3. Bring your left foot back closer to the right foot, back to the beginning position, then gently lift up your right knee.

4. Kick out with the right leg slowly. Be sure to only kick to a height that is comfortable for you.

Alternative: If you have any difficulty balancing with one foot, simply lift your knee up a little, step your right foot forward and touch down on the heel.

Both upper and lower body movements

1. From the Praying Position, slowly turn both hands outwards. At the same time, lift up your left knee slowly, looking to the left at eye level. (Remember, it is okay to do the alternative kick as shown previously.)

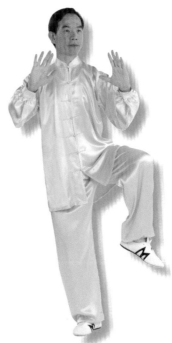

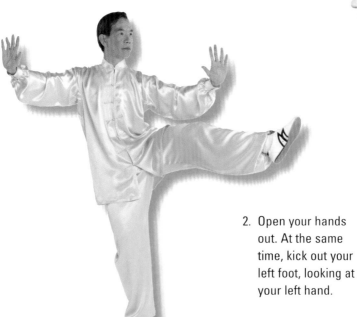

2. Open your hands out. At the same time, kick out your left foot, looking at your left hand.

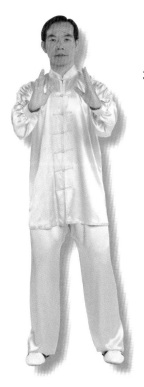

3. Slowly bring your left foot back to the ground and bring your hands back to form the Prayer Position.

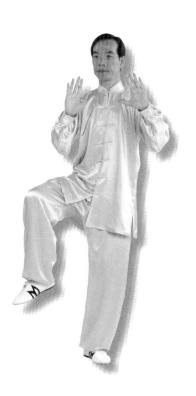

4. Slowly turn both hands outwards. At the same time, lift up your right knee slowly, looking to the right at eye level.

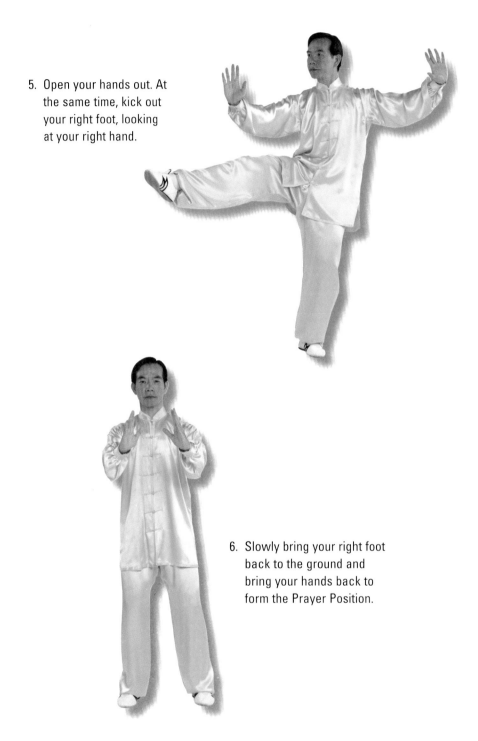

5. Open your hands out. At the same time, kick out your right foot, looking at your right hand.

6. Slowly bring your right foot back to the ground and bring your hands back to form the Prayer Position.

MOVEMENT 8

OPEN AND CLOSE HANDS

Repeat Movement 2.

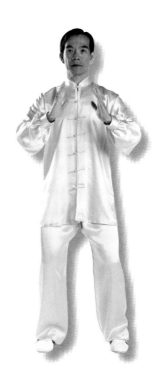

TAI CHI FOR LIFE

Hour for hour, tai chi is probably the most effective exercise to improve your health and wellbeing. You can start — and continue — to improve no matter what your age or physical condition.

Tai chi was created based on nature and harmony. The gentle flowing movements contain inner power that strengthen the body, improve mental balance and bring better health and harmony to people's lives.

More importantly, tai chi helps you to know and like yourself better. This will lead you to health and harmony within yourself and with others.

MOVEMENT 9

WAVING HANDS IN THE CLOUD (RIGHT)

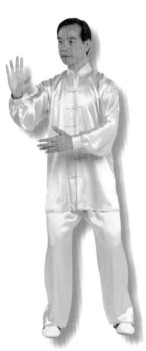

1. Turn slightly to the left, bringing your hands to the left with the right hand on top. At the same time, step out with your right foot.

2. Step your left foot closer, and bring both hands to the right.

3. Turn your right palm out

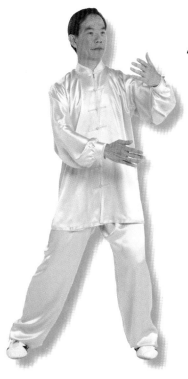

4. Swap hands. Bring them to the left. At the same time, step out with your right foot.

5. Turn your left palm out. Then swap hands and bring them to the right to repeat Waving Hands two more times — making a total of three Waving Hands.

MOVEMENT 10

OPEN AND CLOSE HANDS

Repeat Movement 2.

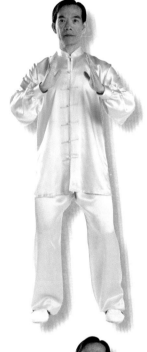

MOVEMENT 11

CLOSING MOVEMENT

1. Gently stretch your hands forward to shoulder height and shoulder-width apart.

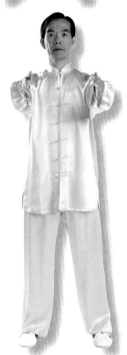

2. As you gently lower your hands, stand up slowly.

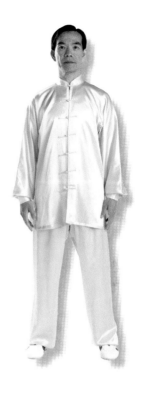

3. Bring your left foot closer to the right foot, back to the starting position. Remain in this position for a few seconds, stay focused and allow your energy to go back to the dan tian.

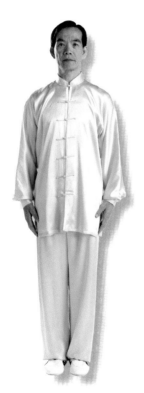

The advanced set

At the centre of the advanced set is Stroking Bird's Tail, which is the theme movement of Yang-style tai chi. It consists of four key techniques and is challenging to learn. Be sure you are quite proficient with the basic set before you start this.

The advanced set combined with the basic set offers a flowing set of forms with an exercise level similar to brisk walking or higher (depending on the height of your stance and how much internal power you use). When doing the advanced set, continue from the basic set's Movement 10 (Open and Close), skip Movement 11, then move on to Waving Hands (left) and continue with the following sequence.

1. Waving Hands in the Cloud (left, x 3)

2. Open and Close Hands

3. Stroking Bird's Tail (left)

4. Open and Close Hands

5. Stroking Bird's Tail (right)

6. Open and Close Hands

7. Waving Hands in the Cloud (right, x 3)

8. Open and Close Hands

9. Closing Movement

MOVEMENT 1

WAVING HANDS IN THE CLOUD (LEFT)

1. Move both hands to the right side of your body. At the same time, step out with your left foot.

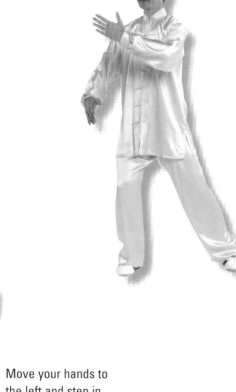

2. Move your hands to the left and step in with the right foot.

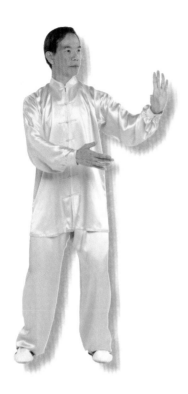

3. Slowly turn your left palm out.

4. Bring your left hand down and right hand up slowly.

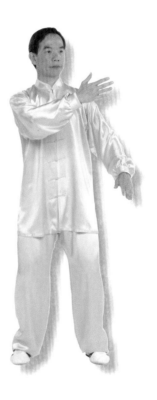

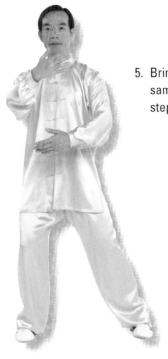

5. Bring hands to the right. At the same time, turn your waist and step out with the left foot.

6. Slowly turn your right palm out.

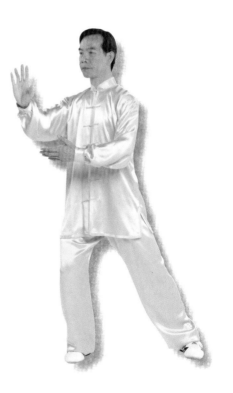

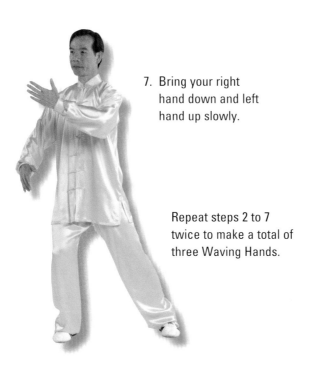

7. Bring your right hand down and left hand up slowly.

Repeat steps 2 to 7 twice to make a total of three Waving Hands.

MOVEMENT 2

OPEN AND CLOSE HANDS

Repeat Movement 2 of the basic set.

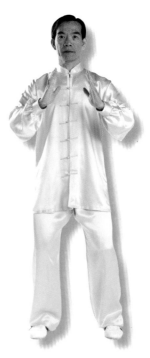

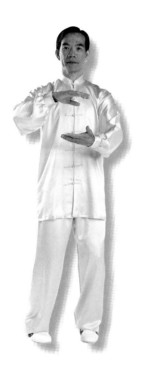

MOVEMENT 3

STROKING BIRD'S TAIL (LEFT)

1. Shift your weight slightly to the left, turning your right toes inwards at 45 degrees. At the same time, move your hands in a curve to end with your right hand up and left hand down, as if you are carrying a ball.

2. Shift your weight back to the right, and step out to the left with your left foot 90 degrees from the front (to 9 o'clock starting from facing 12 o'clock). Move your hands slightly towards each other as though you are gently squeezing a ball.

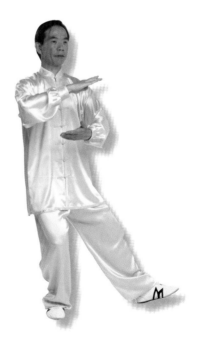

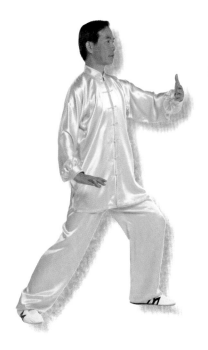

3. Shift your weight forward gradually, making sure not to overbend your left knee — if you look down, you should just be able to see the tip of your toe. (It is better to bend a little, staying well within your comfort zone, rather than doing a deep knee bend.) At the same time, slowly separate your hands, moving your left hand forward to form a semi-circle in front of you, and your right hand next to your hip, with the fingers pointing forward.

4. Shift your weight forward very slightly, and turn your waist, also very slightly, towards the left. At the same time, stretch out both hands, so that your left hand turns to the left with the palm facing out, and your right hand is near your left elbow, with the palm facing up.

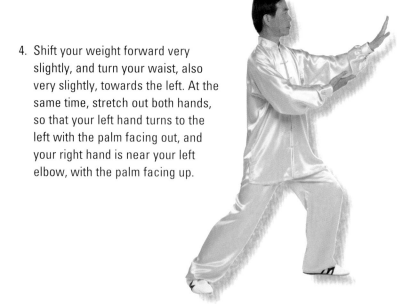

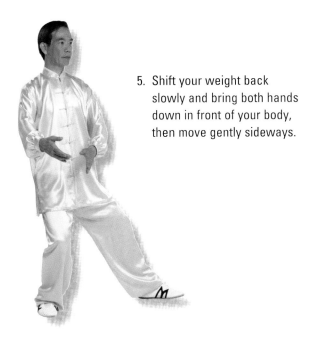

5. Shift your weight back slowly and bring both hands down in front of your body, then move gently sideways.

6. Slowly turn your body to the side. At the same time, move both hands in a gentle curve sideways, so that both your hands are at the right corner, with the right hand at eye level with palm up (looking at the right palm as if you were looking at a hand-held mirror) and the left palm facing down and near the right elbow.

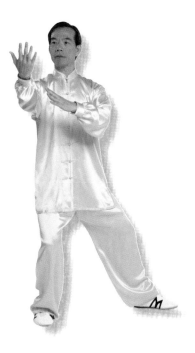

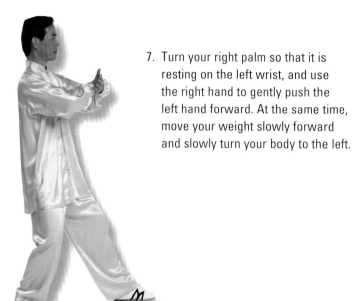

7. Turn your right palm so that it is resting on the left wrist, and use the right hand to gently push the left hand forward. At the same time, move your weight slowly forward and slowly turn your body to the left.

8. Continue to use the right palm to push the left hand forward so that both hands form a semi-circle in front of the chest. At the same time, shift your weight forward slowly.

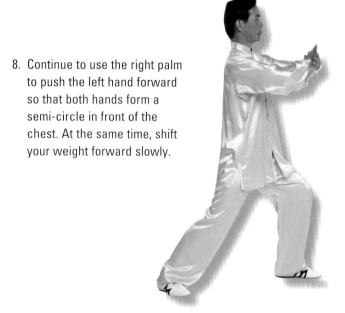

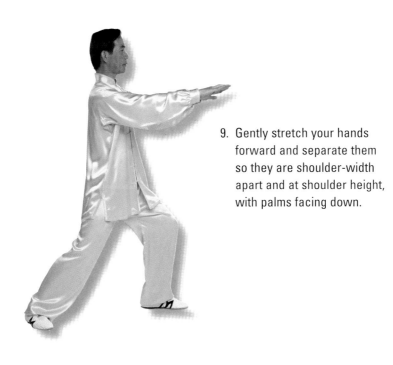

9. Gently stretch your hands forward and separate them so they are shoulder-width apart and at shoulder height, with palms facing down.

10. As you shift your weight back, gently bring your hands back to chest height.

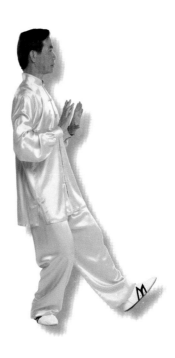

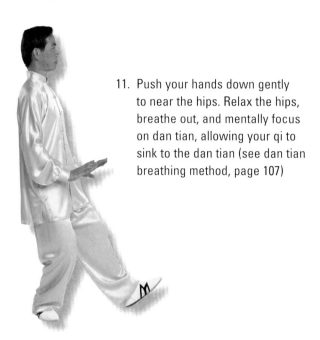

11. Push your hands down gently to near the hips. Relax the hips, breathe out, and mentally focus on dan tian, allowing your qi to sink to the dan tian (see dan tian breathing method, page 107)

12. Gently push your hands forward and upwards in a gentle curve. At the same time, move your weight forward.

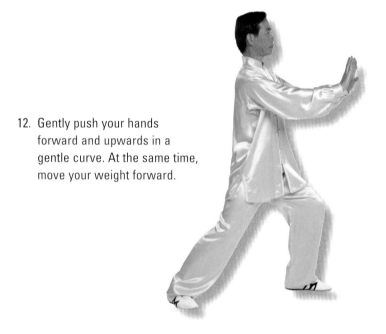

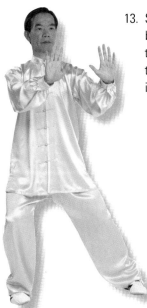

13. Shift your weight back, bringing your hands back, then turn your left toe to face the front so that the left foot is now pointing at 12 o'clock.

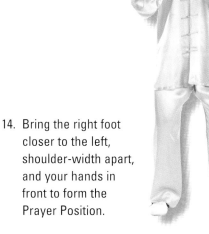

14. Bring the right foot closer to the left, shoulder-width apart, and your hands in front to form the Prayer Position.

MOVEMENT 4

OPEN AND CLOSE HANDS

Repeat Movement 2 of the basic set.

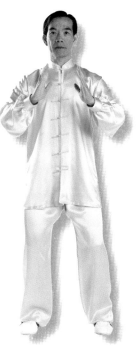

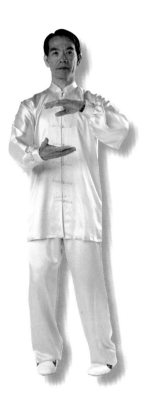

MOVEMENT 5

STROKING BIRD'S TAIL (RIGHT)

1. Shift your weight slightly to the right, turning your left toes inward. At the same time, move your hands in a curve to end with your left hand up and right hand down as if you are carrying a ball.

2. Shift your weight back to the left, and step out to the right with your right foot 90 degrees from the front (pointing at 3 o'clock). Move your hands slightly towards each other as though you are gently squeezing a ball.

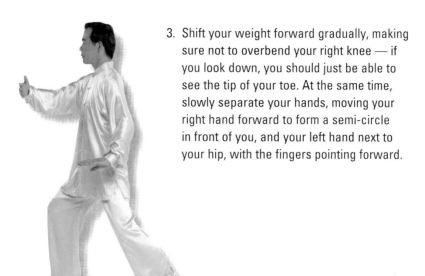

3. Shift your weight forward gradually, making sure not to overbend your right knee — if you look down, you should just be able to see the tip of your toe. At the same time, slowly separate your hands, moving your right hand forward to form a semi-circle in front of you, and your left hand next to your hip, with the fingers pointing forward.

4. Shift your weight forward very slightly, and turn your waist, also very slightly, towards the right. At the same time, stretch out both hands, so that your right hand turns to the right with the palm facing out, and your left hand is near your right elbow, with palm facing up.

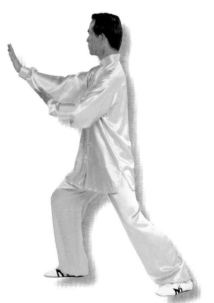

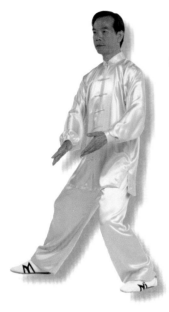

5. Shift your weight back slowly and bring both hands down in front of your body, then move gently sideways.

6. Slowly turn your body to the side. At the same time, move both hands in a gentle curve sideways, so that both your hands are at the left corner, with the left hand on top with palm up and the right palm facing down near the left elbow.

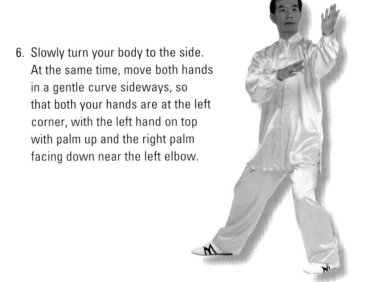

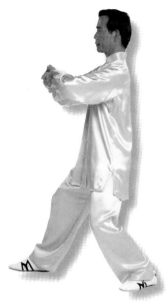

7. Turn your left palm so that it is resting on the right wrist, and use the left hand to gently push the right hand forward. At the same time, move your weight slowly forward and slowly turn your body to the front.

8. Continue to use the left palm to push the right hand forward so that both hands form a semi-circle in front of the chest. At the same time, shift your weight forward slowly.

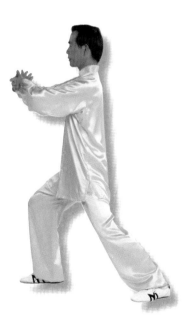

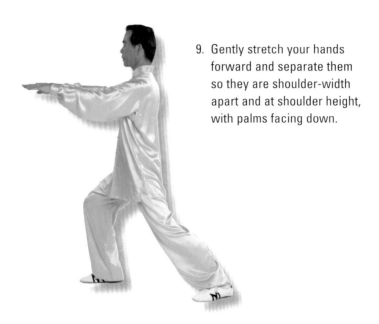

9. Gently stretch your hands forward and separate them so they are shoulder-width apart and at shoulder height, with palms facing down.

10. As you shift your weight back, gently bring your hands back.

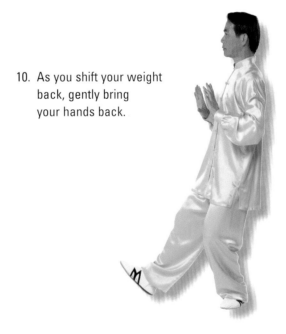

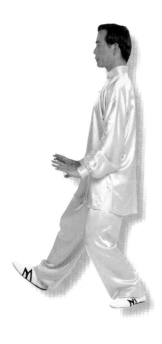

11. Push your hands down gently to near the hips. Relax the hips, breathe out, and mentally focus on dan tian.

12. Gently push your hands forward and upwards in a gentle curve. At the same time, move your weight forward.

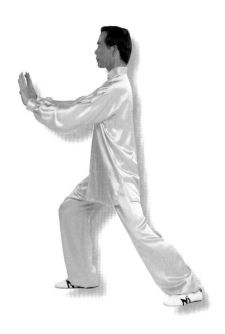

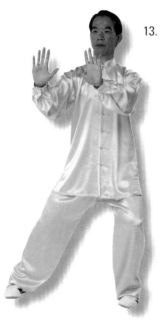

13. Shift your weight back, bringing your hands back, then turn your right toe inwards to face the front pointing at 12 o'clock.

14. Bring the left foot closer to the right, shoulder-width apart, and your hands in front to form the Prayer Position.

MOVEMENT 6

OPEN AND CLOSE HANDS

Repeat Movement 2 of the basic set.

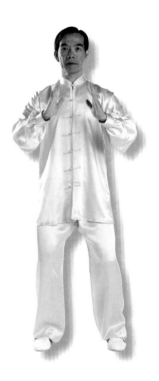

MOVEMENT 7

WAVING HANDS IN THE CLOUD (RIGHT)

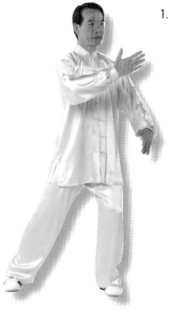

1. Turn slightly to the left, bringing hands to the left with right hand on top. At the same time, step out with the right foot.

2. Step left foot closer, and bring both hands to the right.

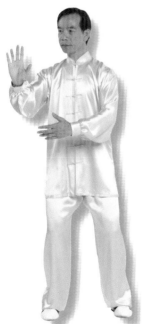

3. Turn your right palm outwards.

4. Swap hands. Bring both hands
   to the left while stepping
   out with the right foot.

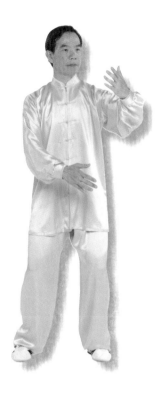

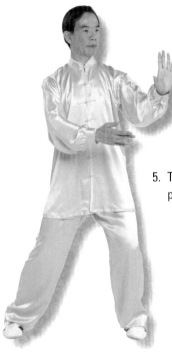

5. Turn your left
   palm out.

6. Swap hands, bring hands to the right. Repeat Waving
   Hands twice to make a total of three times. It does
   not matter if you repeat it more or less times.

MOVEMENT 8

OPEN AND CLOSE HANDS

Repeat Movement 2 of the basic set.

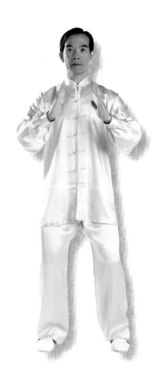

MOVEMENT 9

CLOSING MOVEMENT

Repeat Movement 11 of the basic set.

How to improve your tai chi

After you have learned the program you will have a good foundation of tai chi. Going beyond this is to a higher level will give you more enjoyment and greater health benefits. People learn differently. Some prefer concentrating on one area and others learn by working on different aspects. You can continue to improve on what you've already learned or you can venture out and learn a new set of forms or a new style. Either approach can take you to a higher level, as long as you continue to practice.

Tai chi is not a sport in which you move up in some standardised grading system, nor is it a competitive sport in which one wins and the other loses. In tai chi, the achievement is an intrinsic reward, one that gives you a sense of personal fulfillment as well as the enjoyment of practice and better health.

At a high level, to varying degrees, tai chi tends to become a way of life for the practitioner. Sun Lu-tang, the creator of the Sun style and one of the greatest tai chi masters in history, said that the highest level of tai chi is not about being invincible but is about achieving a deep understanding of the Dao. The Dao is nature. A practitioner will reach the highest level of tai chi when he or she is in harmony within him- or herself and with nature. At the high level of tai chi, it is this internal component that matters most.

It's not necessary to learn more sets of tai chi in order to reach a high level. According to one tai chi teacher, 'Over the last thirty years, I've learned many sets of forms. My greatest improvement came from teaching the simple sets of forms. When I teach how to integrate the essential principles into these simple sets, I demonstrate. And as I demonstrate, I focus on integrating the principles. Through the numerous repetitions, I have found that my understanding of the essential principles deepened each time, and as a result, my level of tai chi and forms improved immensely.'

What is the right way to do tai chi?

Often, tai chi beginners ask, 'Is there only one right way?' If you lived back in the old days, you'd be spending your lifetime seeking out 'the best teacher'. Then, you would devote yourself totally to studying under that person. You'd have absolute faith, and, to you, there'd be only one truth — and one best teacher.

But, of course, there's no such thing as one 'best teacher' and, in any case, limited exposure often ends with limited ability. Learning tai chi today offers a lot more opportunities. How the ancients would have loved to have opportunities to know different styles and teachers before committing to one teacher. Today, we have a better chance to see what works best for us. Seeing the bigger picture can help us to progress.

In Yang style, for instance, you move forwards and backwards by lifting your foot just off the ground and touching down like a 'cat'. In Chen style, you step forward, brushing your foot and often stomping noisily on the ground. So after learning that you should lift your foot up to step forward, it can be strange to then see Chen stylists dragging or brushing their feet on the ground.

'Depress the chest and raise the upper back' is one of the ten essential points by Yang Chen-fu, one of the most famous tai chi masters in history. But what does that mean? Different people interpret it differently. To many, it means relaxing the chest and allowing your qi to reach your back. Many Yang stylists hunch their backs because that is the way they interpret this particular point.

Different styles even have different hand shapes: Yang style uses an open palm, for example, and Chen uses a closed one. Even within one style, you might encounter many variations, and even significant differences.

All this tells us that one style or one person cannot be completely right and everyone else wrong. As there are many roads leading to Rome, so there are many right ways to do tai chi. Minor differences aren't important. The key to improving your tai chi is to understand and integrate the essential principles of tai chi, which are similar in all styles.

Guidelines

It is challenging and fun to continue to strive for a higher level, but it's important to understand that no one knows all about tai chi, nor is it important to be perfect. The enjoyment and benefits come from the experience of practice and progress. Only through regular practice will you truly understand the inner meaning of tai chi as well as receive its great benefits. So make practice a top priority.

Here are four guidelines that will help you to progress whichever way you choose to move on.

Follow the essential principles

Despite the many variations of tai chi, its immense power for improving health and inner energy derives from a set of essential principles. Here are the most important ones. By keeping them in mind as you learn and practice, you'll be able to do tai chi more effectively right from the beginning. To see if you're following these principles, you can use a video camera, a mirror, or work with a friend or instructor.

1. Do your movements slowly, without stopping. Make them continuous like water flowing in a river and don't jerk. Maintain the same speed throughout.
2. Imagine you are moving against a gentle resistance. That will cultivate your inner force (qi). Imagine the air around you is becoming denser and that every move you make is against a gentle resistance — like when you move in water.
3. Be conscious of weight transference. This is important for improving mobility, coordination and stability. Be aware when you transfer your weight and of each step of your weight transference. When you move forward, for example, put your weight on one leg while maintaining an upright, balanced posture; touch down gently with the other heel first, and then place the entire foot on

the ground by gradually putting more of your weight onto that foot.

4. Maintain an upright posture and body alignment. Keep the body straight without creating tension, which can be quite difficult, especially when you start bending your knees. Often, when people bend their knees, the body alignment become distorted. Test yourself, standing side on to a mirror — don't look at the mirror. Bend your knees and look at the mirror now. Is your back in a vertical line to the ground? A good way to keep a good alignment as you do this is to imagine that you are going to sit on an empty chair. Bend both your knees and hip joints. Practice this with the mirror and check yourself every now and then. Once you have achieved good body alignment, your tai chi will improve greatly because qi flows best in the aligned body. Hunching forward will hinder the qi flow, and compromise your balance. Leaning backward will create extra strain to the spine. So try to keep your body upright throughout all movements. Take into consideration different body contours, aim at moving upright gradually and keep well within your comfort zone.

5. Loosen or 'song' the joints. You should relax when you do tai chi — but relax doesn't mean letting your muscles get floppy. Instead, consciously and gently stretch your joints from within, almost like you're expanding your joints internally. Many people mistranslate the Chinese word 'song' as relaxation. This is only half right. 'Song' means both relaxed and loosened. To practice loosening the spine, imagine it's a string, and that you are gently stretching it from both ends. For the lower limbs, bend your knees, crouch and stretch your hips out to form an arch with your thighs. Other upper limb joints will gently expand from within.

6. Focus on your movements, being mindful of where you are and where your body is in time and space. Avoid distractions and focus on what you're doing. Be aware of all the principles mentioned above, but think of them one at a time.

Extend the essential principles

To improve your tai chi, it is essential to progress in four different 'directions': jing, song, chen and huo. These are extensions of the essential tai chi principles. The following repeats some of that information but explores it in different ways.

The four directions complement each other, so you don't need to be completely proficient in one before moving on to another. They also affect each other positively, so that by learning more about one you will improve your understanding of the others. Try working on one direction for a period of at least a few weeks and then move on to another. But come back to each one regularly.

Some of the concepts below might not be clear to you. Don't let that concern you. As you progress further, you'll be able to understand them. In time, as your level of understanding deepens, the words will take on somewhat different meanings. Bear in mind that no one reaches perfection in all four directions — progression is what matters.

Jing

Jing, roughly translated, means 'mental quietness' or 'serenity'. To attain this quietness of the mind, imagine yourself in a tranquil environment such as a shady rainforest. If you do this regularly, you will soon be serene, or quiet from within, and be able to focus on what your body is doing.

Attaining a degree of mental quietness takes time. But once achieved, it will stay with you — the next time you practice, your mind will be able to relocate the same state — and gradually you will be able to move on to an even higher level. Jing improves relaxation and allows you to focus. This, in turn, enhances balance and relieves muscle tension, making your tai chi practice more effective.

The mental quietness of tai chi is different from that of other forms of meditation. While you are serene from within, you are still aware of your environment and able to assess the situation around you at any time — which is essential when you're performing tai chi as a martial art. Although jing might be a more difficult mental state to achieve than, say, meditation, once attained it will help to improve your tai chi but also assist with any crisis in real life. Even just saying the word jing quietly to yourself may help to induce the state.

Song

Song is often translated as 'relaxation', but it means more than that in Chinese, conveying a sense of loosening and stretching out. Imagine all your joints opening, loosening or stretching out gently from within. Take your shoulder joint, for example. If you gently stretch out that joint, you'll feel and most likely see a small dimple on the top of the shoulder. If you tense the shoulder joint, the dimple disappears.

Now apply this technique to other joints. Visualise them loosening. In the upper limbs, loosen your elbows, wrists and finger joints by stretching them out, almost like gently pulling the joint open. In the torso, the loosening should be vertical — visualize your spine as a string that you gently stretch from both ends. For the lower limbs, stretch your hip joints and knee joints gently outwards, so that your crouch forms an arch.

This method of loosening constitutes a type of controlled relaxation, because when you gently stretch your joints you release tension. Song helps your qi flow, builds internal strength and also improves flexibility. It will also enhance jing. Once you develop song, your mind becomes jing as well and, as your mind becomes more jing, your song will improve, thus setting up a positive circle.

Chen

Chen (not the same word in Chinese as the name of the style) means 'sinking'. As you progress in tai chi, you'll come across the term 'sinking your qi to the dan tian'. An area three finger-widths below the belly button, the dan tian is central to everything we do in tai chi as it is the main storage house of qi.

Exhaling facilitates the sinking qi to the dan tian, which in turn keeps your mind jing and loosens up your joints. The feeling of qi differs from person to person but, for most, it's a warm, heavy feeling. As you breathe out, loosen your joints. You should feel a warm, heavy feeling in your dan tian. That's the feeling of sinking your qi. If you don't feel this initially, don't worry. Continue to practice the form and, as you improve, you'll eventually feel the qi in the dan tian and learn how to sink it. It does not matter whether you feel the sinking of qi, thinking about it as described will facilitate the qi cultivation.

Chen enhances stability, song, and qi cultivation. Awareness of the dan tian will strengthen the internal structures of your body, improve your inner strength and strengthen your spine.

Huo

Huo means 'agility'. Being strong, having powerful qi and being in a good mental state are essential, and these attributes are even more effective with better agility. Agility comes from regular practice, using the proper body posture, weight transference, control of movements, loosened joints and strong internal strength. Agility aids qi cultivation and improves flexibility.

Use these strategies for improvement

We've made it clear that to improve your tai chi you must understand the tai chi principles and practice regularly and with awareness. Now let's look at some other methods that will help you improve your skills. Some of these will work more effectively for some learners than for others, but they should help most people.

Getting beyond the plateau phase

In his book *Mastery*, the well-known Californian martial art expert George Leonard describes the 'plateau phase'. He explains that learners go through phases. In between each quantum leap of technical advance, there's a long plateau phase in which improvement is slow and not obvious. This phase is necessary for absorbing knowledge and skill before rapid advancement can happen.

A typical learning curve therefore looks like this:

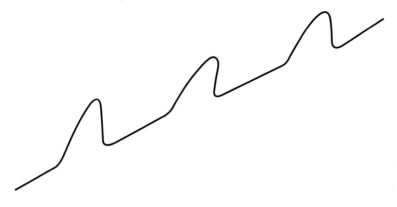

Steep rises are separated by wide plateaus. Impatient students become bored and disappointed during the plateau phases and often drop out. In tai chi, plateaux and steep rises are yin and yang. The former is storing energy and the latter is delivering energy. You need to store energy before you can deliver it. Like tai chi, this is nature. In the long run, being aware of and learning how to enjoy the plateaux will help you persist and make significant progress. Learning about flow can help you enjoy the plateau phases more.

Getting your flow going

Flow occurs when a person is so absorbed or so fully engaged in an activity that he or she becomes 'lost in time'. It often happens when an athlete performs at his or her best, or when an artist paints a masterpiece. Athletes sometimes call it being 'in the zone'. Whether you are doing a job, hobby or sport — or tai chi — if you are fully engaged, you are more likely to be 'in flow'.

After years of studying many thousands of people, Professor Mihaly Csikszentmihalyi, a director of psychology and education at the University of Chicago and the author of *Finding Flow*, has found a close connection between enjoyment and flow: people whose lives are fulfilled and serene are more often in flow. He also found that it is possible to increase the flow experience. These findings are well supported by other experts.

You can work to increase your flow. If you can enjoy what you're doing, you know you will do better. More flow also means better tai chi.

Three main factors can induce flow:

1. Having a clear goal or goals.
2. Receiving immediate and relevant feedback.
3. Matching your goals to your skills.

'Goal' in this case means a short-term goal. For example, your goal for one round of practice could be to move smoothly or it could be simply to remember the movements. You'll know right away if you have remembered the movements correctly and if they're smooth. In other words, you will get immediate and relevant feedback.

Matching your goals to your skill level will result in greater satisfaction. For example, if you're a newcomer to tai chi and unfamiliar with the moves, trying to do them smoothly could be too challenging and thus lead to excess stress; on the other hand, if you're experienced in tai chi, you may already be doing your moves smoothly, so this goal may offer no challenge at all, which could lead to boredom. In other words, if the skill required to attain a goal is beyond your capacity, you are likely to get stressed, which would prevent you from entering the flow state; and if a goal is too easily achieved, you will get bored and are unlikely to experience flow.

In tai chi, we aim to integrate body and mind, which can take you to a mental state similar to flow. As your tai chi improves, you'll be in flow more often. More flow will bring you more enjoyment, more enjoyment will drive you to practice more, and more practice will result in more flow. The end result is a healthier and more fulfilled life.

Feeling good naturally

The human body resonates with nature, and tai chi follows the rhythms of nature, so practicing tai chi will make you feel in tune with nature and in harmony with yourself. Try to work towards nature's flow and rhythm in your practice.

Learning new skills

Learning something new often stimulates people to try harder. We've observed that with students, some of whom have travelled thousands of kilometres to attend our annual one-week tai chi workshops. At the end of the workshops, they demonstrate what they have learned. The sparkle in their eyes from these demonstrations shows very clearly their pride and pleasure. So whether you're learning a new set of forms or reaching the depth of the forms, you are learning new skills. Recognise and feel the excitement of that.

Helping people

Many tai chi practitioners around the world teach tai chi. Most do it for the enjoyment they get out of helping people improve their health and quality of lives. Helping others is a powerful motivator, an integral part of human nature. By being of value to others, we gain great self-esteem and fulfilment. So try to teach whenever you can. Teaching is also one of the best ways to improve your own skills.

Getting the habit

Humans are people of habit. We like following routines. Set a regular time daily to practice. And once you get into that habit, you'll find that your mind and your body will demand it.

Feeling better

Many scientific studies have shown the health benefits of tai chi. By practicing it, numerous people have made significant improvements to their health and the quality of their lives. And the point is, they've done it themselves. They have taken control of improving their own life situations. The health benefits, and the pride they feel in their achievements, drive people to practice and improve their tai chi.

Using mind power

Tai chi is an internal art, which means that you have to use your thinking ability. This is a big part of what makes tai chi so interesting. Evidence shows that the mind is like the body — you either use it or lose it. Regular use of your thinking ability improves it and prevents disease such as dementia or Alzheimer's. Keep using your mind when you are practicing. Analyse your moves. What is the intrinsic purpose of the move? Does it make good sense? Does it feel comfortable? Does it feel balanced? Is it consistent with tai chi principles? Does it give you a stronger feeling of qi? Is it safe? Analysing your own tai chi is the best way to gain deeper understanding and make improvements.

Using mind power also means being open. If you're fixed on one idea and close your mind to others, then you can't take in anything else. On the other hand, an open mind is ready to take in or absorb new knowledge, and you will progress.

Absorbing

Your food must be digested to make it useful to your body. You also have to digest tai chi until it gets inside your body, into your bones and becomes a part of you. When you learn a new technique or form, you should try to practice it until you digest it well before acquiring new skills. Only after digestion can you expand the skill.

Using self-guided imagery

The unconscious mind has strong control over us. To improve your tai chi, try using self-guided imagery, which is an excellent technique to train your unconscious mind. (See an article by Dr Yanchy Lacska and Dr Paul Lam in *Tai Chi for Beginners and the 24 Forms*, 2006.)

Letting go

This was summed up perfectly in an inspiring talk by Sheila Rae, a tai chi and qigong teacher: 'There comes a point in our practice when we must learn to let go of the form, the perfectionism, and of the ego.'

The very act of letting go implies that we are in possession of something. When we apply this concept to tai chi, we understand that without learning and practicing the form, we do not posses tai chi awareness. But this awareness is not just a product of perfected moves and steps. Although good form is vital to the overall experience, it is not the end goal for the serious practitioner.

As we begin tai chi, the ego helps us to see what we can achieve. It is powerful, fun and exciting. But like anything we practice to learn — such as piano, dance, even cooking — there comes a time when we must let go of trying to follow prescribed patterns and let the art move through our souls. It's at this point, by letting go of the form, that we can realise the true meaning for our study — which is to integrate the tai chi principles into our daily lives. Yes, we've heard that before and understand the importance of that aspect of tai chi training: but we must even let go of that, otherwise we might judge others who are not using tai chi principles in their lives. Try letting go in life so that the principles can apply to life — and then your life will influence your tai chi. If we can surrender in movement, the form will express the surrender.

If we constantly train to perfect its moves, we can't realise the true bliss of doing tai chi. By letting go of the form, wonderful connections can happen. First, the moves connect together effortlessly, then we can connect to the true essence of blending with our environment, with others and with the universe itself. We must learn to let go of the form to find the connectedness we are seeking.

Work with a teacher

Sooner or later, if you are to progress to a higher level, you'll realise that you will need a teacher. Face-to-face instruction from a suitable teacher can enhance your tai chi immeasurably. On the other hand, an unsuitable teacher can set you back. People we know have given up tai chi because they've had unsuitable teachers. So take your time to find a teacher with whom you resonate well and who will meet your needs.

A good teacher should guide you, no matter what stage you're at in tai chi. If the teacher starts by saying, 'Everything you've learned thus far is all wrong, you've wasted your time,' look for another teacher. There is not just one way in tai chi, there are many good ways.

If you live in a fairly large community, chances are you won't have much trouble locating teachers. Ask friends for recommendations. (You can also consult Dr Lam's website at www.DrPaulLam.com, which includes a list of instructors worldwide.) Make contact with the teachers. Find out what style they teach. Do they take someone at your level? What's the charge? Ask if you can observe a class.

When you visit a class, watch the students, and if possible talk to them. Do they seem interested? Enthusiastic? Do they ask questions and get satisfactory responses? Are their objectives similar to yours? Are there regular students? A British tai chi instructor, Margaret Brade, provided this fine explanation of why she thought so highly of her teacher: 'I still went back to him as he had some magic for me — and many others. It is hard to capture in words what someone has that makes thirty-plus people turn up twice a week, week after week — all those instructors who have come after him (he has now retired) have not managed it and people still constantly talk of Bruce.'

Does the teacher care about injury prevention? Are warm-up and cooling-down exercises part of the teaching? Is the teacher more interested in martial art or health?

Finding a teacher might be more difficult for those in small towns. You might have to take workshops or use instructional DVDs and books rather than attending classes. However, in addition to regular home-based classes, many excellent tai chi teachers travel to give courses. You can often find out about these courses and workshops online.

MAKING THE MOST OF CLASSES

Once you decide on studying with a teacher, you can get more out of your classes by keeping the following suggestions in mind.

- Always try to understand your teacher. Open your mind and be receptive. Show respect, which will help you connect better with your teacher.

- Be prepared for corrections, negative feedback and even criticism. Remember that many teachers are particularly hard on talented students. If you see criticism in that light, you can treat it as a compliment for being a talented student!

- Prepare for your lessons. That way, you'll get the most out of them. Find out what the next lesson will be on and get ready for it. That way you'll learn more.

There may come a time when you feel you've learned as much as you can from your teacher. Perhaps it's time for you to make a change. Don't feel guilty. Each teacher has something different to offer. Why not take advantage of that fact? Simply let the teacher know in a respectful way, show your appreciation and be honest about why you are leaving.

In the tai chi world, it's not uncommon to come across teachers who teach in a 'traditional manner'. Many such teachers expect students to learn simply by following them doing the forms, and they don't provide any instructions, hands-on assistance or individual attention. They may even discourage communication or be negative about a student's progress. Some traditional teachers also demand total loyalty: they don't allow you to be instructed by another person or even use books and DVDs. Nowadays, however, these teachers are becoming rare.

This isn't to say that traditional-style teaching is all bad. Many traditionally oriented teachers have much to offer. Whether you opt for this kind of instruction depends on your understanding, tolerance, how you learn best and whether you have any choice.

PART IV

RESOURCES

Resources

Tai Chi

WEBSITES SUPPORTING TAI CHI FOR HEALTH PROGRAMS

www.taichiforhealthcommunity.org
Tai chi for Health Community, a non-profit organisation, based in USA and dedicated to bring tai chi to as many people as possible for health improvement.

www.betterhealthcc.com.au
Better Health Tai Chi Chuan, Inc., a non-profit organisation based in Australia, aims to create a friendly and interactive environment for all members to grow through tai chi.

www.ageconcernstockport.org.uk
Age Concern is the largest charity provider in the United Kingdom, working with, and for, older people. Age Concern in Stockport provides support and classes for Tai Chi for Health programs.

www.rheumato.org
Korean Association of Muscle and Joint Health provides support, workshops for Tai Chi for Health instructors' training, research and classes across South Korea.

www.taichiforhealth.com
This website contains tai chi information, discussions, lists of Tai Chi for Health instructors worldwide, and up-to-date products from Dr Paul Lam.

BOOKS

Dr Paul Lam and Judith Horstman, *Overcoming Arthritis*, Dorling Kindersley, Melbourne, 2002.

Dr Paul Lam, *Teaching Tai Chi Effectively*, East Acton Publishing, Sydney, 2006.

Dr Paul Lam and Nancy Kaye, *Tai Chi for Beginners and the 24 Forms*, Limelight Press, Sydney, 2006.

Simplified Taijiquan, China Sports Series 1, compiled by China Sports Editorial Board, Beijing.

Sun Lu Tang, *Xing Yi Quan Xue, The Study of Form: Mind Boxing*, translated by Albert Liu, compiled and edited by Dan Miller, High View Publications, 1993.

The Essence of T'ai Chi Ch'uan: The Literary Tradition, translated and edited by Pang Jeng Lo, et al, North Atlantic Books, Berkeley, CA, 1979.

Barbara Davis, *The Taijiquan Classics*, North Atlantic Books, Berkeley, CA.

Bill Douglas, *The Complete Idiots' Guide to Tai Chi and Qigong*, Alpha Books, New York.

Martin Lee, et al, *Ride the Tiger to the Mountain – Tai Chi for Health*, Perseus Books Reading, Massachusetts, 1989.

Chia, Mantak and Juan Li, *The Inner Structure of Tai Chi*, Healing Tao Books, Huntington, NY, 1996.

Compiled by Morning Glory Press, *Yang Style Taijiquan*, Hai Feng Publishing

Co, Hong Kong, 1988.

Compiled by Zhaohua Publishing House, Hong Kong, *Chen Style Taijiquan*, Hai Feng Publishing Co, 1984.

Taiji: 48 Forms and Swordplay, China Sports Series 3, China Sports Editorial Board, Beijing.

Douglas Wile, *Cheng Man-Ch'ing's Advanced T'ai-Chi Form Instruction*, Sweet Chi Press, Brooklyn, NY, 1985.

Dalai Lama and Daniel Goleman, *Destructive Emotions, How We Can Overcome Them*, Bantam Books, New York.

Dr Stephen T Chang, *The Complete System of Self Healing: Internal Exercises*, Tao Publishing.

Isabelle Robinet, *Taoist Meditation, The Mao-Shan (Shang-ch'ing) Tradition of Great Purity*, State University of New York Press, New York.

MAGAZINES

T'ai Chi, the international magazine of T'ai Chi Chuan
Wayfarer Publications, PO Box 39938, Los Angeles, CA 90039-0938, USA
www.tai-chi.com

Qi, the journal of traditional Eastern health and fitness
Insight Publishing Inc, PO Box 18476, Anaheim Hills, CA 92817, USA
www.qi-journal.com

TAI CHI ASSOCIATIONS

www.taichiaustralia.com
Tai Chi Association of Australia: promotes tai chi in Australia.

www.betterhealthtcc.com.au
Better Health Tai Chi Chuan, Inc., a non-profit organisation.

www.worldtaichiday.org

World Tai Chi & Qigong Day, the biggest event in tai chi worldwide, organised by Bill Douglas.

www.taichiamerica.com
Tai Chi America: provides a multimedia learning resource and archive for all interested in tai chi chuan and chi kung.

www.taichiunion.com
Tai Chi Union in Britain.

DVDS

Dr Paul Lam has worked with teams of experts to produce several series of tai chi DVDs, from introductory teach-yourself series for health to the advanced series designed to expand skills. Titles include:

Tai Chi for Arthritis (English, Chinese, French, Spanish, German and Italian versions)

Tai Chi for Arthritis II

Tai Chi for Diabetes

Tai Chi for Osteoporosis

Tai Chi for Older Adults

Tai Chi 4 Kidz

Tai Chi for Beginners (English, Chinese, French, Spanish, German and Italian versions)

Qigong for Health

Tai Chi: The 24 Forms

The 32 Forms Tai Chi Sword.

Contact Tai Chi Productions (www.taichiproductions.com) for the intermediate and advanced series.

Diabetes

BOOKS

Diabetes and You: The Essential Guide, Diabetes Australia, Canberra, 2001.

Guide to Exercise, National Heart Foundation, available from National Heart Foundation, Hutt Street, Adelaide, SA.

Driving and Diabetes — covers the legal and practical requirements for driving with diabetes.

American Diabetes Association, *Complete Guide to Diabetes*, 4th edition, American Diabetes Association, 2005.

Jennie Band-Miller, Kaye Forster-Powell and Stephen Colagiuri, *The New Glucose Revolution*, Hodder, Sydney and Auckland, 2002.

Neal D Barnard, *The Reverse Diabetes Diet: Control Your Blood Sugar, Repair Insulin Function and Minimise Your Medication — Within Weeks*, Rodale, New York, 2007.

Darryl E Barnes, with the American College of Sports Medicine, *Action Plan for Diabetes, Your Guide to Controlling Blood Sugar*, Human Kinetics, USA.

Beyond the Basics: Lifestyle Choices for Diabetes Prevention and Management, Canadian Diabetes Association, 2007.

Beyond the Basics: Meal Planning Resource, Canadian Diabetes Association, 2006.

Ann Holzmeister, *Diabetes Carbohydrates and Fat Gram Guide*, 3rd edition, American Diabetes Association.

Anne Daly, Linda M Delahanty and Judith Wylie-Rosett, *101 Weight Loss Tips for Preventing and Controlling Diabetes*, American Diabetes Association.

Sheri R Colberg, *The 7-Step Diabetes Fitness Plan*, Marlowe and Company, USA, 2006.

EATING AND COOKERY BOOKS

The following are available from the Diabetes Australia:

- *Enjoyable Eating:* a simple guide to healthy eating.

- *Enjoyable Eating Recipe Folder:* a set of healthy recipes in a binder to which you can add.

- *Enjoyable Eating on a Budget:* a guide to healthy eating on a budget.

Diabetes and Heart Healthy Cookbook contains healthy recipes created by the combined work of the American Diabetes Association and the American Heart Association. With cardiovascular disease number one on the list of diabetes-related complications, this is a must-have cookbook for people with diabetes and people with heart disease.

Take 5: a guide to preparing healthy food using five basic ingredients.

Alan Borushek, *Calorie Counter Plus Carbohydrate and Salt Guide*, (or similar), available from pharmacies or drugstores.

DIABETES ORGANISATIONS AND SUPPORT

Australia

Diabetes Australia
Diabetes Australia is a not-for-profit, member-based organisation. It provides advocacy and access to many services for people with diabetes. There is an office in each state where you can access videos, books and products, as well as education. A national magazine, published four times a year, provides information about managing diabetes and the latest research. Some state branches also run local support groups and web pages. There is a yearly membership fee. Phone 1300 136 588 to find out more or access the website at www.diabetesaustralia.com.au.

The National Diabetes Services Scheme (NDSS)
The National Diabetes Services Scheme supports people with diabetes by

providing access to reliable and affordable supplies and services, thereby assisting with self-care. The NDSS started in 1987 and is funded by the Australian government. Diabetes Australia looks after the scheme on the government's behalf.

Registration is free and the only requirements to register are that you have been diagnosed with diabetes, that you live in Australia and that you hold or are eligible to hold a Medicare card.

People who are registered with the NDSS can access a range of government-approved products including:

- subsidised testing strips
- free syringes and pen-needles if you require insulin
- subsidised insulin pump consumables for eligible registrants
- a range of information services.

The NDSS has agents in all capital cities.

State/Territory	NDSS Agent
ACT	Diabetes Australia, ACT
NSW	Diabetes Australia, New South Wales
NT	Healthy Living, NT
QLD	Diabetes Australia, Queensland
SA	Diabetes South Australia
TAS	Diabetes Tasmania
VIC	Diabetes Australia, Victoria
WA	Diabetes Australia, Western Australia

Each NDSS agent manages a number of sub-agents which, in most cases, are located in local chemists. A list of sub-agents in your state or territory is available at www.ndss.com.au/sub-agents. Alternatively, you can also phone the NDSS during business hours from anywhere in Australia for the cost of a local phone call on 1300 136 588 and your call will be redirected to the nearest NDSS agent.

Medicines and supplies
Supplies can be obtained through:

National Diabetes Services Scheme (NDSS)
This scheme is the cheapest way to buy blood- and urine-testing strips and other supplies. Registration can be arranged through Diabetes Australia.

Private and hospital prescriptions
A prescription is required to purchase all diabetes medications. Urine- and blood-glucose monitoring strips can also be obtained through pharmacies if you have a prescription.

Supplies available without a script
Blood-glucose testing strips can be purchased, but at higher prices than from the NDSS or with a prescription.

Meters
These can be bought from Diabetes Australia, some hospital clinics and some pharmacies. Make sure you understand how to use and maintain the meter and what you are to do if the blood-glucose values are too high or too low.

Websites
There are a number of useful websites that you can access.
www.diabetesaustralia.com.au
Diabetes Australia

www.diabetesaustralia.com.au/multilingualdiabetes/index.htm
Diabetes Australia Multilingual resources

www.realitycheck.org.au
Reality Check: support for young adults

www.diabetescounselling.com.au
Advice and counselling

www.adea.com.au
To find a accredited diabetes educator
www.daa.asn.au
To find an accredited practicing dietitian

www.apodc.com.au
To find an accredited podiatrist

www.austroads.com.au
Assessing fitness to drive

www.carersaustralia.com.au
Carers Australia

www.jdrf.org.au
Juvenile Diabetes Research Foundation

Social and economic issues
For long-term stress or unresolvable social issues (family problems, financial), seek professional help. Discuss with your GP or diabetes healthcare team.

Canada
Canadian Diabetes Association
The the Canadian Diabetes Association offers a wide range of educational and information programs and services to help you learn more about your condition and meet others living with it. The association has a useful website at www.diabetes.ca and branches throughout the country.

New Zealand
Diabetes New Zealand
Diabetes New Zealand is the national organisation that acts for people affected by diabetes. It encourages local support, raises awareness of diabetes, educates and informs people, and supports research into the treatment, prevention and cure of diabetes. See www.diabetes.org.nz for information on services, latest research, news and events.

United States of America
The American Diabetes Association
The association is the nation's leading nonprofit health organization and

provides diabetes research, information and advocacy. Founded in 1940, the American Diabetes Association conducts educational programs in all 50 states, reaching hundreds of communities. Its website, www.diabetes org, contains a great deal of useful information about prevention, nutrition, weight loss programs and current research on diabetes.

National Call Center

The American Diabetes Association runs a national call centre, which provides information on diabetes and on its programs and events, as well as support services. The service is available in English and Spanish.
1-800-DIABETES

United Kingdom

Diabetes UK

Diabetes UK is the largest organisation in the UK working for people with diabetes, funding research, campaigning and helping people live with the condition. Its website is www.diabetes.org.uk.

Diabetes glossary

A1c: Haemoglobin, the red protein in blood, with glucose chemically bound to it. Also called *glycosylated haemoglobin* or *HbA1c* ; it represents the average blood glucose level over the last 120 days, a very useful measurement of how well controlled your diabetes is.

Arteriosclerosis: The walls of the arteries are damaged. Fat and calcium build up inside the walls and may slow the blood flow. Also called *atherosclerosis* and *hardening of the arteries*.

Carbohydrate: A nutrient in food which provides energy for the body. Carbohydrates include sugars, starches and fibre (roughage) found in foods such as fruit, milk, cereals, starchy vegetables and bread.

Coronary artery: A blood vessel which carries blood to the muscle of the heart.

Glucagon: A hormone produced in the pancreas. It causes stored glucose (glycogen) to move from the liver into the blood stream to be used as energy. Glucagon can be given as an injection if hypoglycaemia causes unconsciousness.

Glycosylated haemoglobin: See *A1c*.

Glycosuria: The presence of glucose (sugar) in the urine.

Haemoglobin: The red-coloured iron protein that carries oxygen in red cells.

Insulin Dependent Diabetes Mellitus (IDDM): Now known as type 1 diabetes. Also called *Juvenile Onset Diabetes*.

Ketone: Chemical substance formed by the breakdown of body fats. It can be dangerous in large amounts.

Ketonuria: The term used to describe ketones in the urine.

Juvenile Onset Diabetes: Now known as type 1 diabetes. Also called *Insulin Dependent Diabetes Mellitus (IDDM)*.

Mature Onset Diabetes: Now known as type 2 diabetes. Also called *Non Insulin Dependent Diabetes Mellitus (NIDDM)*.

Microalbuminuria: Leakage of small amounts of protein (albumin) into the urine. An early warning of kidney damage.

Nephropathy: Kidney damage.

Neuropathy: Nerve damage.

Non Insulin Dependent Diabetes Mellitus (NIDDM): Now known as type 2 diabetes. Also called *Mature Onset Diabetes*.

Oral hypoglycaemic agent: Diabetes tablets used to treat type 2 diabetes.

Retinopathy: Damage to the blood vessels at the back of the eye.

Type 1 and type 2 diabetes: The two main forms of diabetes. In type 1, no insulin is being made; type 2 is characterised by insulin resistance and insufficient insulin to overcome the resistance.

Acknowledgements

We are grateful to Diabetes Australia for allowing us to reproduce sections of their invaluable diabetes manual, *Diabetes and You: The Essential Guide* (2nd edition, 2002), and to the Diabetes Centre of The Queen Elizabeth Hospital for permission to reproduce parts of the Diabetes Education series.

We would like to thank our publisher Lisa Hanrahan, who has exceptional energy and enthusiasm, and the editor, Mary Trewby, who put colour and clarity into the text.

— Paul Lam and Pat Phillips

Many people have contributed significantly and it is impossible to name you all. Thank you all to my tai chi friends, students and colleagues who have inspired and supported this program. Diabetes New South Wales, and especially Lillian Jackson, its director of programs, and Alan Barclay, research manager, have been exceptionally supportive and helpful.

I am particularly grateful to the instructors and students of my tai chi school, Better Health Tai Chi Chuan Inc. Thanks also go to the manager, Anna Bennett, and her staff at Tai Chi Productions, and to my USA distributor Sheila Rae. I am thankful for your dedication to my tai chi vision by making it possible for me to spend time on this book. My family has also contributed significantly to this project — thanks for your support and love.

— Paul Lam